Learning the Brainstem

Learning the Brainstem

Edison K. Miyawaki, M.D.

Copyright © 2019 by Edison K. Miyawaki, M.D..

Library of Congress Control Number:		2019900430
ISBN:	Hardcover	978-1-7960-1028-2
	Softcover	978-1-7960-1027-5
	eBook	978-1-7960-1026-8

All rights reserved. No part of this book may be reproduced or transmitted in any form or by any means, electronic or mechanical, including photocopying, recording, or by any information storage and retrieval system, without permission in writing from the copyright owner.

Any people depicted in stock imagery provided by Getty Images are models, and such images are being used for illustrative purposes only.
Certain stock imagery © Getty Images.

Print information available on the last page.

Rev. date: 01/15/2019

To order additional copies of this book, contact:
Xlibris
1-888-795-4274
www.Xlibris.com
Orders@Xlibris.com
790295

Contents

1 Introduction 1
2 Three Choices 2
3 The Diencephalic-Mesencephalic Border 10
4 Just at the Superior Colliculi 14
5 At the Levels of CN III Complex 21
6 They Stare at Me 27
7 Rostral Pons 36
8 Properly in the Fourth Ventricle 44
9 Beyond Brazis 50
10 On the Facial Colliculus 54
11 What About the Weakness? *"L'hémiplégie alterne"* 67
12 Folded Grey Mass 72
13 Oblivious to Ocular Lateropulsion 80
14 Canonical Medulla 87
15 A Note on Brainstem Vasculature 94

References 101

1.

Introduction

Nothing worth really knowing is easy to learn, but there are productive strategies.

This short book, intended for interested medical and neuroscience students, compiles tactics that I've used over years of teaching human brainstem anatomy. I'll assume familiarity with a basic neurological examination before we begin. I've noticed that medical students now learn in clinics and hospitals during their first year of school; so be it. That early exposure to patients and their problems demands better teaching from the elders amongst us, myself most certainly included.

Another thing to mention at the start: I know that some students consider themselves purely visual learners, but if the reader anticipates that there will be excellent diagrams in what follows, then I'd ask that person not to be unduly disappointed.

The written word aids an ability to visualize anatomy in the mind's eye. Such is my approach.

In evaluating a patient, one doesn't want to consult an illustration at the bedside. You'd seem like a tourist with a map.

To achieve knowledge like that of a local: I'll attempt it.

2.

Three Choices

When it comes to the localization of a brainstem lesion, to keep things simple, a person has three choices. The problem could be in the medulla, pons, or midbrain.

I've taught many students who, if presented a random axial section of brainstem, can't tell whether she or he looks at a slice of pons, midbrain, or medulla. It's OK. The problem has to do with how we teach the subject, that's all.

Even if you just guessed, you'd have a one-in-three chance of being correct. The odds in a true-false question are better, yes. All the same, a one-in-three chance isn't bad. Midbrain, medulla, or pons: those are the possible answers. Just choose one. If you're right, then you figure out why you were correct. If wrong, then you ascertain how you went astray from brainstem reality.

You've started to learn our subject.

*

Off my shelf, I pull a worn copy of *Localization in Clinical Neurology* (Brazis et al., 1985). It's a book I consulted *a lot* during my training in the 1980's. It has 21 chapters, ten of which address either cranial nerves III through XII; or the midbrain, pons, and medulla; or the topic of coma. Roughly half of the book, then, deals with the very limited amount of neurological space that comprises a brainstem, which is about three inches in length. (The coma chapter deals heavily with brainstem, even if coma often results from bihemispheric dysfunction only.)

I turn to chapter 14, "The localization of lesions affecting the brainstem," which is only 14 pages long, including notes. The old highlighting in my copy has faded–note to self: yellow ink is evanescent, as memory can be. The author wastes no time; he starts with syndromes of the medulla oblongata (the medulla) on his first page.

If you're like the way I once was, you seek the shortest, best rendition of facts, names, and tidbits–all of which you must assimilate quickly. You have zero patience for encyclopedic performances. As much as I still like chapter 14, there's a problem with the method: it's full of facts ready for memorization. It reads like a 14-page shopping list of stuff to get at the store.

As said, if someone has any question about anything having to do with the brainstem, it's a matter of three basic options. You know that short list already. Now we get to work.

We'll consult two early papers, both decades old (I'll provide the references later). The plan is to think through the authors' problem by entertaining our three possible answers.

*

They wanted to solve a "particular puzzle": "*the localization of a lesion that could cause both pyramidal and cerebellar signs in the same limbs* [my italics]."

Here's a synopsis of the first case in their series.

A 44 year-old man, whose past medical history included (perhaps) a touch of high blood pressure, noticed while walking one afternoon that his right knee was "wrong." He felt that the right leg could buckle under him. He sat down to have a cigarette; as he lit it, his right hand overshot the mark. He was able to walk to the doctor's office, which wasn't far away ("200 yards"). Turning the pages of a magazine in the waiting room was difficult, due to incoordination in his right, presumably dominant hand. He was examined. All of the above happened within 50 minutes of onset of his difficulties. As he put his shoes back on, after the examination, he noticed clearing of all his symptoms. But they returned five minutes later.

(I have to ask: he was just 200 yards away from the doctor's office? And the office actually added him to the schedule? But I digress.)

His vital signs were notable for a blood pressure of 138/104. On general medical examination, he was overweight, but there were no reported abnormalities. The pertinent findings were all neurologic. He was alert without a speech disorder. Specifically, he was not dysarthric. His visual acuity and visual fields were normal. The optic discs were normal, as were his pupils, including their reaction to light. Eye movements were full, except that, on left lateral gaze, there was horizontal nystagmus with a fast component to the left. Optokinetic nystagmus was diminished with leftward moving targets. His face was symmetrical; hearing was normal, as was his swallowing. His tongue was not weak.

He was weak in the distal right leg; right ankle and toe dorsiflexion were poor. Otherwise he was strong. Sensation was normal throughout to the primary modalities, but he described that his right hand felt "swollen." There was reflex asymmetry only in the legs: the right knee jerk and ankle jerk were brisk compared to the left; the right toe was clearly extensor, the left flexor.

Appendicular coordination, gait, and Romberg were all abnormal. I'll quote the findings verbatim:

> The right arm and leg showed a severe intention tremor . . .. On the finger-nose test wild oscillatory movements caused the patient to strike himself in the face. The patient could not use the right hand for eating. Abnormal rebound was easily demonstrated. On holding the arms out the right deviated laterally. On the heel-knee test there was a most severe dysmetria and the right thigh tended to fall laterally although weakness could not be demonstrated. . . . Walking was unsteady

and the right leg was dragged with toe scraping and circumduction . . .. On the Romberg test the patient toppled backwards and to the right.

Bearing in mind that the title of this monograph is *Learning the Brainstem*, it wouldn't serve a teacher's purpose to present, off the bat, a case that's not a matter of brainstem localization. I know my students well enough to predict that a handful would pounce and protest, "but it's not necessarily a brainstem problem." The authors acknowledge as much: "If first we set aside for the moment the proposition that the syndrome is the result of a supratentorial lesion, how might an infratentorial lesion explain the symptoms?" The **tentorium cerebelli** is dura mater that "intervenes" between the cerebral and cerebellar hemispheres (Nolte, 1999); that tentorium is the upper border of the posterior fossa, wherein the brainstem, infratentorially, . . . is.

So, we've got three choices for localization in the infratentorial brainstem.

One approach is to improve the odds. Can we eliminate just one option to get us to a 50-50 chance?

*

Let's think about the eyes first, since nystagmus was the first reported finding, aside from his high-ish blood pressure and his body's perhaps over-heavy mass. His mental status was normal. He was "intelligent," in fact. All seemed fine in talking with him, but . . .

A practical thing to do is to notice what's working fine, long before one obsesses over some alleged direction-fixed or unidirectional nystagmus (leftward beating on leftward gaze), never mind the oddity of their optokinetic nystagmus finding.

The eye movements were full. Can we surmise that cranial nerves III, IV, and VI, and their brainstem nuclei, and perhaps the white-matter connections between them . . . were all intact? If you ran with that hypothesis, then you might exonerate midbrain, the location of the nuclei of cranial nerves III and IV, as well as pons, the location of cranial nerve VI nucleus, from affliction.

Note to self: cranial nerves assigned lower numbers are located higher up–they are more rostral. (Cranial nerve I is most rostral, but it has little to do with the brainstem; cranial nerve II has to do with the upper brainstem insofar as some of its fibers project *to* brainstem.)

Cranial nerve nuclei III and IV are mesencephalic, in the midbrain.

By the time you get to two major cranial nerve V nuclei–there's a sensory one and motor one in the pons–you're (guess what?) in the upper/rostral pons.

Could we say that the localization of the 44 year-old man's problem must be in the medulla, by exclusion of the midbrain and pons, because the eye movements were full?

*

> **RULE #1**, which might be called the rule of rules and the mother of a scientific approach to anything: whenever in doubt or, especially, when you are certain beyond doubt, assume that you are wrong (that you are null); then assimilate data to prove or disprove your null hypothesis.

*

There was a left-beating nystagmus elicited only in left lateral gaze. Presumably, it wasn't present in primary gaze (looking straight ahead); not present, either, with the eyes in right lateral gaze. What does it mean? The authors don't help much: "[It's] a somewhat indefinite finding but one which should not be dismissed too readily." Are we already confused? Can we say, for now, that something might not be normal with gaze in the lateral plane?

In part, gaze in the lateral plane has to do with the lateral rectus muscle, associated with cranial nerve (CN) VI, whose nucleus is below that of CN V, but still in pons. There was even a problem with the eyes looking at leftward moving targets in a test to elicit optokinetic nystagmus. Is it perfectly safe to eliminate pons from consideration? We might subtract a bit from our earlier hypothesis: if CN III and IV seem to be OK, can we take midbrain off our list at least?

*

RULE #2, related to RULE #1 (as important as RULE #1): whatever you do, keep working the problem.

*

The last sentence raises a reasonable question: what *is* the problem? His right leg is wrong. And he couldn't light his cigarette. It all happened quickly, just two football fields away from his doctor.

Now let's translate the findings on examination into simple sentences.

FIRST (BIG) OBSERVATION: *He was weak in the distal right leg; right ankle and toe dorsiflexion were poor. Otherwise he was strong.* TRANSLATION: He had a isolated right foot drop.

SECOND OBSERVATION: *There was reflex asymmetry only in the legs: the right knee jerk and ankle jerk were brisk compared to the left; the right toe was clearly extensor, the left flexor.* TRANSLATION: There were upper motor neurons signs in the right leg and foot.

THIRD (MAJOR) OBSERVATION: *The right arm and leg showed a severe intention tremor. On the finger-nose test wild oscillatory movements caused the patient to strike himself in the face. The patient could not use the right hand for eating.* TRANSLATION: No wonder he couldn't light his cigarette. I'll bet that getting the cigarette to his lips wasn't easy, either. A task with a target was a problem for him, because of shaking or shakiness. More on his right leg in a moment.

FOURTH: *Abnormal rebound was easily demonstrated. On holding the arms out the right deviated laterally.* TRANSLATION: One assumes a relationship between these findings and the third observation.

FIFTH: *On the heel-knee test there was a most severe dysmetria and the right thigh tended to fall laterally although weakness could not be demonstrated.* TRANSLATION: How can a person walk with this problem? The authors already told us about a right leg tremor, but this sounds different, maybe.

SIXTH: *Walking was unsteady and the right leg was dragged with toe scraping and circumduction.* TRANSLATION: Are we talking only about his foot drop (see first observation)? With a foot drop, the toe would indeed scrape the ground, despite all circumducting attempts to prevent that from happening.

Unsteady walk? What does that mean?

SEVENTH: *On the Romberg test the patient toppled backwards and to the right.* TRANSLATION: Originally, Moritz Heinrich Romberg's test (he taught in Berlin in the mid-19th century) had to do with neurosyphilis. Let's assume that our patient doesn't have neurosyphilis.

*

Summary of where we are this moment, point by point: 1. Teacher says this is not a case of neurosyphilis, so that's off the list; 2. We tentatively excluded the midbrain as a localization–which leaves us with pons vs. medulla; 3. The patient has a weak distal right leg and something really wrong with the right arm and leg when either of them move, especially towards a target; 4. We know for an absolute fact that there's a combination of pyramidal and cerebellar signs, because the very first thing we read about the case was the authors' interest in *the localization of a lesion that could cause both pyramidal and cerebellar signs in the same limbs.*

I'm not trying to be flippant–and we'll return to the above case in chapter 9. For now, I draw attention to the fact that cerebellar and pyramidal tracts are closest to each other physically/anatomically, and therefore can both be affected by one acute and discrete lesion, either in the midbrain or pons. Cerebellar and pyramidal tracts are comparatively far apart in the medulla. Earlier in our discussion, we excluded the midbrain, more or less. So, by a kind of primitive logic, could we say that the lesion localization in our 44 year-old gentleman must be pontine?

The papers used in this chapter are Fisher and Cole, 1965 and Fisher, 1978. The syndrome is an ataxic hemiparesis. The brainstem localization is left pons, although ataxic hemipareses can result from supratentorial lesions.

3.

The Diencephalic-Mesencephalic Border

Since the brainstem as a whole is such a small territory, the argument could be made that all structures in it are close to each other by definition. That's true, but all things are relative. In anatomy lab, if you take a thin slice of any part of the brain, structures visible on one surface often look very different on the reverse side; sometimes, they just disappear. The thickness of the slice could be much less than an inch. In brainstem especially, a great deal changes visually and anatomically in the space of millimeters. Relations are invaluable, however (what's next to what, in detail, at roughly 6-8x magnification, using your mental lens). In the chapters that follow, we'll concentrate on things close to each other at various levels of midbrain, pons, and medulla—in that descending (rostral to caudal) order.

We'll describe axial (transverse) sections, with a proviso.

*

RULE #3: Think three dimensionally.

*

An immediate application of Rule #3 takes the form of a question: is there midbrain above the level of cranial nerve (CN) III complex?

(Answer: yes.) The question invites another: what's above the midbrain? Which leads to yet one more: what's the boundary between midbrain (also known as mesencephalon) and the diencephalon immediately above and contiguous with it?

*

> **RULE #4**: More a convention than a rule, we'll apply the following to all our axial sections: ventral brainstem is *below* dorsal brainstem. (If you look at MR or CT images of brain, ventral brainstem is *above* dorsal brainstem.)

*

THE DI-MESENCEPHALON. The diencephalon, as we recall from developmental anatomy (so long ago, for me), consists of four strata best visualized early in embryonic life: from dorsal to ventral, they are the *epithalamus* (destined to become the pineal gland and habenular nuclei, among other things), *dorsal thalamus* (which will develop into thalamus and all its nuclei), *subthalamus* ("a continuation of the midbrain tegmentum"), and *hypothalamus* (Kahle, 1986). So, honestly, is there a clear division between midbrain/mesencephalon and diencephalon, if the midbrain tegmentum "continues" into subthalamus, among whose structures is the subthalamic nucleus of Luys?

I'm obsessing about the border for two reasons. First, the di-mesencephalic boundary is discrete, based on gene expression in development: PAX6 is found in telencephalon and diencephalon down to the di-mesencephalic boundary, at which border (only after crossing it, heading inferiorly) there's expression of genes like En1, En2, and PAX 2 (Nakamura, 2001). All the above genes are implicated in the differentiation (the "regionalization") of mesencephalon as opposed to prosencephalon—the latter includes both diencephalon and telencephalon. Increasingly, anatomy isn't just dissection and photomicrography anymore, since genes govern anatomic relations.

Second, if you happen to consult good neuroanatomy atlases (e.g., DeArmond et al., 1989), you can't help but notice that *oblique axial sections result in images in which structures at different vertical levels appear in the same picture.* For example, thalamic nuclei can show up in axial sections of the most rostral midbrain, given the vertical proximity of thalamus (and other diencephalic structures) and the mesencephalon. All of thalamus is diencephalic, and the midbrain is mesencephalic—which is to say, they're different, but they're neighbors. The same can be said of hypothalamus and mesencephalon.

Imagine a midbrain section *above* the level of CN III nuclear complex, and you'll visualize both the **red nuclei** and two other round nuclear structures dorsal to the red nuclei—all four are close to the midline. The dorsal ones must be thalamic; you're visualizing the circular centromedian nuclei of thalamus which are dorsal and superior to the red nuclei. If you're not familiar with any thalamic nuclei, then perhaps there's incentive for me to write a different monograph about them. But the point is not to be confused or befuddled if presented with a non-canonical image of midbrain. (By "canonical" in this context, I refer to a midbrain image in which we clearly see the midline, shark's-tooth, or "V"-shaped appearance of cranial nerve III complex, about which more later).

At the di-mesencephalic transition, you might visualize a wispy white-matter tract crossing the axial midline from side to side. We're not referring to the monstrously large corpus callosum connecting *hemispheres* with each other. At the current, very rostral level of *midbrain*—above the level of the superior colliculi—there are really only two options as to what the thing is: the habenular commissure or the posterior commissure, both of epithalamic origin. The posterior commissure is much larger than the other. But the thin **habenular commissure** is interesting, because you might notice that there's a bit of gland (not white matter) in the midline, just dorsal to it. That's the pineal gland, which is epithalamic/diencephalic, not mesencephalic.

The rostral, dorsal mesencephalon, which we're discussing and which derives from a dorsal (or alar) plate, differentiates into an "**optic tectum**," a term most familiar to vertebrate neuroanatomists (Sato et al., 2004). The optic tectum has cellular lamination similar to that seen in visual neocortex, and the optic tectum is a terminus of optic tract in many animals, but not in humans (Carpenter and Sutin, 1983). In other words, you could envision the very rostral midbrain and the superior colliculus, which we're about to introduce, as preeminently and phylogenetically *sensory and visual.*

I haven't discussed the ventral bulk of midbrain at this level (people refer to a midbrain tegmentum, but the etymology confuses me; as in the word "integument," the root of *tegmentum* refers to a "cover"; anatomists talk about how the brainstem "covers" the ventricular system, but I think it's an odd term nevertheless). **Red nucleus** resides in midbrain tegmentum; ventral to red nucleus, there's also **substantia nigra**; dorsolateral to the substantia nigra is the lens-shaped **subthalamic nucleus of Luys**, which is of diencephalic origin (it derives from the stratum called subthalamus).

There are the fiber tracts which connect globus pallidus and thalamus via the upper midbrain, including an **ansa lenticularis** (*ansa*, Latin = loop) and a **lenticular fasciculus**. The ansa lenticularis and lenticular fasciculus will converge into the **thalamic fasciculus**, one of whose destinations is the **zona incerta**, a ventral continuation of the reticular nucleus of thalamus (Haubenberger and Hallett, 2018). All the fiber tracts just mentioned illustrate how midbrain "continues" into subthalamus and thalamus.

Note to self: there are surgical interventions for the treatment of tremor that target the zona incerta of thalamus. If a lesion is placed, for example, in or near the left zona incerta, a reduction in tremor will manifest in the contralateral (right) hemibody. If somebody didn't have a tremor, but suffered a stroke in left zona incerta, would tremor result? Dunno, but, if a tremor appeared, it would be contralateral to the side of the lesion.

I haven't discussed the bulk of midbrain at this level, because I'm waiting for the first evidence of the **quadrigeminal plate** and, in association with it, the posterior commissure.

4.

Just at the Superior Colliculi

Let's move just a bit inferiorly, to the rostral border of the superior colliculi. Nieuwenhuys et al. (2008) cite the dorsal, ventral, and lateral boundaries of our new axial section:

> The border of the mesencephalon with the diencephalon is set caudal to the *posterior commissure* dorsally and caudal to the *mammillary bodies* ventrally. . . . Laterally, it [the midbrain] follows the caudal border of the optic tracts, where the pes pedunculi [cerebral peduncle] emerges on the ventral surface. The geniculate bodies and the pulvinar of the thalamus are located lateral to the rostral mesencephalon.

Despite its textbook authority, the description disorients me. Didn't we just say that the posterior commissure is epithalamic in origin–i.e., above the midbrain? The mammillary bodies belong to posterior hypothalamus, also diencephalic. It won't suffice to say that diencephalon and mesencephalon live on discrete floors of a building. It's not that simple.

Try a thought experiment. Think about a cone. Invert it (apex or vertex pointing down), as if you held an empty ice-cream (sugar) cone. Now imagine an oblique conic section that creates an ellipse rather than a neat circle at the top. We're interested only in the upper/dorsal part of the ellipse—the location, in other words, of the rostral tips of the two **superior colliculi** and a **pretectal area** ("before," ventral, and superior to superior colliculus).

The largest transverse white matter tract that you see at this level is the posterior commissure, which appears very early in the developing human brain, at about ten weeks' gestational age.

The cone in our hand is a three-dimensional shape. What's around it neuroanatomically?

Answers, in terms of anatomic relationships, at the level of the uppermost midbrain:

> VENTRALLY: actually, NOTHING except the cerebrospinal fluid of the interpeduncular fossa (the space between either crus cerebri or cerebral peduncle or pes pedunculi). The mammillary bodies of hypothalamus are also located in that interpenduncular fossa.
>
> DORSALLY: actually, NOTHING, except for the cerebrospinal fluid of the quadrigeminal plate cistern.
>
> LATERALLY: The answer *depends*. Dorsolaterally, there are grey structures symmetrically on either side, because thalamic nuclei (especially, the medial and lateral geniculate bodies) drape over the sides of the midbrain . . . only dorsolaterally. Ventrolaterally, optic tracts wrap themselves around the cerebral peduncles on either side.

Note the physical proximity of these structures, which we've identified so far:

posterior commissure;

pretectal area;
superior colliculi (homologous to the vertebrate optic tectum);
optic tracts; and
thalamic nuclei, in particular, the **lateral geniculate bodies**.

In experiments dating to the 1930's, stimulation of posterior commissure, pretectal area, superior colliculus, optic tract, and areas near but not in the lateral geniculate bodies all produced bilateral pupillary constriction. One might think that either an isolated pretectal lesion or a precise lesion in posterior commissure should disrupt a consensual light reflex, but it appears that only major midbrain damage in pretectal area and posterior commissure *together* impairs expected bilateral pupillary constriction when light is presented to one eye (Carpenter and Pierson, 1973).

We haven't reached an axial section that includes any obvious cranial nerve nucleus, yet we have already discussed much about eyes. We teach that the direct and consensual light response is a reflex whose connections are mesencephalic (optic tract to pretectal area to posterior commissure, without cortical connections).

By comparison, we say that accommodation, otherwise known as the near reflex, involves projections to and from visual cortex. The projection *from* cortex goes *to* midbrain–but where in midbrain? Answer: very high in it, perhaps specifically in rostral superior colliculus in both accommodation and active fixation (Ohtsuka and Nagasaka, 1999).

We talk about saccade generation originating in frontal cortex, in the frontal eye fields, but how often do we think about how the rostral mesencephalon, especially the superior colliculi, might also be responsible for getting eyes to look at certain targets and not others? Hikosaka et al. (2000) beautifully discuss that visual—and maybe not just visual—maps of the world converge in the superior colliculi, and that visual search and saccades were functions that emerged in evolution with the establishment of cortico-superior collicular connections.

In discussing eyes in all five instances (light reflex, accommodation, active fixation, saccade generation, visual scanning), the rostral mesencephalon is like a funnel through which many visual pathways necessarily pass.

*

POSTERIOR COMMISSURE AND THE UPPER AQUEDUCT OF SYLVIUS (CEREBRAL AQUEDUCT). In the upper middle of midbrain at this level sits the cerebral aqueduct, ventral to posterior commissure. Grey matter (**periaqueductal grey**) surrounds the sides of the aqueduct. Once I see the posterior commissure, I know the cerebral aqueduct is ventral to it. Period.

The opposite is not true: if you see the cerebral aqueduct, it doesn't mean that the posterior commissure is necessarily above it. At other levels, the periaqueductal grey encircles the aqueduct completely.

We're now in a position to organize our thinking about the midbrain in general. I think of the midpoint of the cerebral aqueduct in midbrain and rostral pons as part of a side-to-side border between up/dorsal and down/ventral in brainstem.

I'm oversimplifying. There's debate over whether a division between basal and alar plates exists as high as the midbrain (Mastick and Easter, 1996). Lower in the brainstem, particularly in the medulla, we can point to a sulcus (described by Wilhelm His, Sr.) that divides alar and basal plates, but no such landmark exists in midbrain. Yet we can roughly group nuclei above/dorsal and below/ventral to aqueduct in midbrain.

We divide into alar/dorsal and basal/ventral based on sensory and motor nuclei, *respectively.* If we think about the ventral or dorsal location of white-matter tracts or of cranial-nerve fascicles, we'll get confused, especially further down in the brainstem. Alar/dorsal *nuclei* are sensory; basal/ventral *nuclei* are motoric. I can't call it a law; it's just a serviceable principle.

DORSAL/ALAR/SENSORY NUCLEI. Above/dorsal to the cerebral aqueduct, we have the superior colliculi.

*

But what's to be said about these structures, from medial to lateral, on both sides of periaqueductal grey, *just at the level* of the aqueduct:

nucleus of Darkschewitsch and
interstitial nucleus of Cajal.

We'll add:

rostral-interstitial nucleus of the medial longitudinal fasciculus (MLF).

All three are close to each other and to the MLF (yes, MLF is present above the level of CN III nuclei); all structures abut the periaqueductal grey on either side.

Fibers arising from all three nuclei enter the posterior commissure. All three nuclei are, in some sense, sensory, insofar as they receive vestibulocerebellar input and somatosensory information about the position of the head and neck in space. But no anatomist would comfortably call the nuclei of Darkschewitsch, interstitial nuclei of Cajal, and rostral-interstitial nuclei of MLF purely sensory, given the "pre-motor" or "accessory oculomotor" role of all three in the control of eye movements (for a representative discussion, see Fukushima, 1987).

I'll abide by my organizing principle: dorsal to the posterior commissure and to the cerebral aqueduct are the **superior colliculi** ("**optic tectum**"). Those are sensory nuclei just as the lateral geniculate body of thalamus is a sensory nucleus. In fact, the superior colliculi are multisensory, because they integrate more than visual afferent information. Stimulate a right superior colliculus: eyes (conjugately), head, and neck turn to the left. Nauta and Feirtag (1986) talk about how, late at night, if you heard a mosquito, your head orients/turns in the direction of the buzzing intruder: the (multisensory) superior colliculus is involved even in that darkness.

*

Lateral to the cerebral aqueduct, we encounter white-matter tracts:

central tegmental tract (a visible portion of the reticular formation, about which we will have a bit to say, but not now),
spinothalamic, and medial lemniscal tracts.

Very laterally, we're already outside of mesencephalon, because we see medial and lateral geniculate bodies of thalamus.

VENTRAL/BASAL/MOTOR NUCLEI. We see **red nucleus**—"red," because in fresh brain dissections, it looks pink, which is to say iron-reddish. Then there are motor tracts ventral to red nucleus, specifically the three portions of the (ventral) crus cerebri or cerebral peduncle, including, medial to lateral: a **frontopontine tract**, so-called Arnold's bundle, heading inferiorly to pontine nuclei; a central third of the crus which contains corticospinal fibers, many of which will form the pyramid in medulla; and a lateral third of the crus which contains a **temporopontine tract**, so-called Türck's bundle, also headed to pontine nuclei.

The hard-to-miss red nucleus is a defining ventral motor nucleus of the rostral mesencephalon.

The **rubrospinal tract** arises from it, but it's also the terminus of some fibers from contralateral deep cerebellar nuclei.

Ventral to red nucleus, but dorsal to the crus cerebri (its three parts), are the **pars compacta** and **pars reticulata** of the **substantia nigra**. At the level we now discuss, we're below the subthalamic nucleus of Luys, which is no longer visible.

The black, neuromelanin-containing cells of the pars compacta differ from neurons in the pars reticulata. Reticular neurons behave physiologically like pallidal neurons in the globus pallidus pars interna. Compacta neurons are dopaminergic, related to a nigrostriatal pathway that will pass into a **median forebrain bundle** (also known as the medial telencephalic fascicle) medial to the **central tegmental tract**, which we identified previously, en route to the corpus striatum (Moore and Bloom, 1978).

I'd draw attention to the often overlooked, *other* dopaminergic **ventral tegmental area of Tsai**, which is dorsomedial to both parts of substantia nigra and ventral to red nucleus in the interpeduncular midline. Its axons, also via **medial forebrain bundle**, project widely to prefrontal cortex with effects that are beyond the scope of this monograph to describe (for an introductory discussion, see Goldman-Rakic, 1999).

Note to self: red nucleus on one side deals with contralateral hemibody (a left lesion results in right-sided findings in the body). Why? By the time you see the (left) red nucleus, cerebellar fibers have already crossed from (right) contralateral deep cerebellar nuclei. But: most axons from the pars compacta of the substantia nigra project to *ipsilateral* corpus striatum via the homolateral median forebrain bundle. The pars compacta is an extrapyramidal, motoric nucleus. Also: ventral tegmental area projects to ipsilateral cortex (Coenen et al., 2018). Learning which tracts cross the midline and which ones don't causes pain for students universally, I know. I wrote a monograph on the subject, called, perhaps ironically, *The Crossed Organization of Brains*. The organization isn't always crossed (Miyawaki, 2018a).

Cortico-ponto-cerebellar projections (the bundles of Arnold [medial] and Türck [lateral]) reside on either side of pyramidal-tract fibers in the cerebral peduncle. The **red nucleus** hovers dorsal to the cerebral peduncle.

Could an acute, unilateral lesion at this level result in a combination of ataxia and hemiparesis in the contralateral hemibody? If you argue "yes," then how do you to explain the *isolated* foot drop in the case from chapter two?

5.

At the Levels of CN III Complex

The plural is intentional: it's a simple fact that the large CN III complex occupies midline vertical space from the moment we visualize it through all axial sections down to the CN IV nucleus, which has been described as "a small caudal appendage of the oculomotor nuclear complex" (Carpenter and Sutin, 1983).

*

    RULE #5. Find the cerebral aqueduct. If you don't find it, you're not in midbrain.

Please don't misread the rule. There's cerebral aqueduct in the rostral pons as well. The rule only says that there's cerebral aqueduct in midbrain. If you see fourth ventricle, you're not in midbrain.

*

    DORSAL/ALAR/SENSORY NUCLEI. Having applied **RULE #5**, I notice that there's periaqueductal grey all around the aqueduct, but there's no posterior commissure, because we're now below it.

    I apply the principle that nuclei dorsal to/above the level of the aqueduct are sensory. Aside from the **superior colliculus**, there's another sensory nucleus of note, the **mesencephalic nucleus of CN V**, located along the lateral edge of the periaqueductal grey. It's curious for being a dorsal root ganglion inside brainstem parenchyma. Fibers arrive there by way a **mesencephalic tract of CN V**; its afferent information relates to proprioception of the teeth and "the force of the bite" (Carpenter and Sutin, 1983).

VENTRAL/BASAL/MOTOR NUCLEI. We'll concentrate on CN III complex, but we first re-acknowledge white matter tracts that we encountered in the previous axial section, all lateral to red nucleus:

> **central tegmental tract** (a visible portion of the reticular formation, superior to the red nucleus), and, laterally, the **spinothalamic and medial lemniscal tracts**.

Very (dorso) laterally, we're already outside of mesencephalon, because we see medial geniculate body of thalamus; lateral geniculate body has passed out of our field of view.

*

Oculomotor nucleus (we'll discuss just one side of CN III nuclear complex) resides beneath/ventral to the cerebral aqueduct at the ventral margin of the periaqueductal grey. It contains motor neurons that innervate the following muscles:

> medial rectus (MR)
> inferior rectus (IR)
> *contralateral* superior rectus (*contralateral* SR)
> inferior oblique (IO)
> levator palpebrae (LP)

In addition, the parasympathetic Edinger-Westphal nucleus sends preganglionic fibers that synapse at the ciliary ganglion in the orbit: it's involved not only in the control of pupillary constriction (via action of the pupillary sphincter), but also accommodation and blood flow to the ciliary muscle (the latter responsible for changing the shape of the lens in the near reflex). There's both a preganglionic Edinger-Westphal nucleus and a "centrally projecting" Edinger Westphal nucleus–the latter contains a neuropeptide transmitter called urocortin; its central projections aren't entirely clear–perhaps to hypothalamus, the serotonergic dorsal raphe, and even spinal cord (May et al., 2008).

The CN III nuclear complex has subnuclei that are discrete in the vertical space (the ensuing discussion follows Ngwa et al., 2014). There's value in knowing about the location of subnuclei, because you improve your understanding about eye movements in both the vertical and horizontal planes.

*

MR subnucleus first. Just a moment ago, we created a list; there's an intentional and anatomical order to it, from rostral to caudal:

MR, IR, contralateral SR, IO, LP.

Begin, rostrally, with MR subnucleus. Actually, MR subnucleus in humans is present at all axial levels of CN III complex; there are subdivisions of MR subnucleus. But along with the Edinger-Westphal nucleus, at the most rostral extent of the CN III complex *is* a MR subnucleus. Why does this high location make sense?

We've alluded to accommodation or the near reflex, and, at the risk of insulting the intelligence, at very least we know that in accommodating, both eyes adduct at the same time. We've mentioned that rostral superior colliculus or perhaps the pretectal area (what some people call a supraoculomotor area) may be involved in the cortically mediated act of accommodation. A powerful, excitatory vergence input gets both eyes to adduct; we must assume that there's concurrent decrease in firing of the muscle yoked to MR–i.e., a decrease in firing rate of lateral rectus, a muscle we haven't discussed yet (Büttner-Ennever, 2006). MR subnucleus is rostral, as are locales that mediate the brainstem pathways involved in accommodation.

There's an issue, however. The Edinger-Westphal sub-nucleus at this very rostral level contains urocortin (centrally projecting), and is not strictly pre-ganglionic/parasympathetic. The clearest visualization of parasympathetic Edinger-Westphal nucleus happens some millimeters below where we are (at which level we see all CN III extraocular subnuclei together, in the "canonical" section which depicts CN III's full "V" or shark's tooth shape). But preganglionic Edinger-Westphal neurons are diffusely present in the midline CN III complex, even when we can't point to the parasympathetic subnucleus itself.

*

MR and IR subnuclei together. The next subnucleus we encounter is IR. When we see MR and IR subnuclei together, anatomists also identify an unpaired, midline "nucleus Perlia" (it's yet another CN III subnucleus; Richard Perlia described it in 1889). Nucleus Perlia was once thought to be involved in convergence, but later studies haven't confirmed that hypothesis. These days, some people think that it's involved in upgaze.

MR and IR subnuclei are present together in all subsequent caudal sections.

A primary action of IR in the vertical plane is depression of the eye, especially but not only in abduction. But when I think about the near reflex (or if I just look at my own nose, crossing and depressing my eyes to do so), I intuit that the anatomical proximity of MR and IR subnuclei makes sense. Someone will ask about the role of superior oblique, but we haven't arrived at its nucleus yet. (In any event, looking straight down involves *both* IR and superior oblique muscles.)

MR, IR, IO, and *contralateral* SR subnuclei together. At the next caudal level, all CN III subnuclei involved in control of its associated extraocular muscles are present in one axial section.

I've discussed the grouping of IR/IO/contralateral SR in a previous short book, *The Crossed Organization of Brains*. It's vain of me, but I'll cut and paste what I wrote; the subject matter is what happens in both eyes when a quick, corrective saccade happens:

> . . . in a run we take one random day, with one footfall, there's a pothole we didn't expect. It's an irregular

pothole. A foot gets caught in an oblique way, casting us in an oblique direction, but, mercifully, we don't fall. The run continues to our satisfaction, without injury.

As foot meets pothole, I envision events having occurred within just a few milliseconds: unilateral firing of the rostral interstitial nucleus of the MLF, say, on the left, then immediate activation of the following, all on the same side of the midline (on the left): subnuclei of inferior oblique, inferior rectus, [contralateral] superior rectus, *and* the left trochlear nucleus [which innervates contralateral superior oblique]. The result, with short latency between nuclear discharge and muscle action involving the eyes: a corrective saccade involving the left inferior oblique and inferior rectus acting on the left eye, and an equal saccade of contralateral superior rectus and the superior oblique acting on the right eye (Miyawaki, 2018a).

There's sense in the grouping of IR, IO, and *contralateral* SR subnuclei. Right eye intorts and left eye extorts, all at once (Büttner-Ennever, 2006).

The central caudal nucleus. The most caudal of the CN III subnuclei is an unpaired nucleus which contains motor neurons that innervate the levator palpebrae on either side. It's not clear why, but motor neurons in the central caudate nucleus are mainly inhibited by GABA-ergic neurons located at the level of the posterior commissure.

Imagine a combination of findings, as Henri Parinaud introduced them in 1883: a main finding is an upgaze paresis in both eyes; the paresis could be bad enough that the eyes look downward in the primary position ("sun setting" eyes); in attempting upgaze, the eyelid widens so that you see a good bit of white sclera above the limbus of the iris (Collier's sign, a failure in normal inhibition of central caudal nucleus); also in attempting upgaze, sometimes there's a nystagmus in which the fast phase moves towards the midline in both eyes, a convergence nystagmus; yet accommodation is poor (in fact, the pupils look dilated, and they stay that way). People refer to a "syndrome of the cerebral aqueduct"; it's a good term, because multiple levels of CN III complex must be involved to produce its constellation of signs.

6.

They Stare at Me

In my first year teaching neuroanatomy, I regularly identified the CN IV (trochlear) nuclei as part of the midline structure called CN III nucleus. I made the mistake consistently. Since then, I've been fascinated by young teachers' errors (and those of old academics, too; I still err often). The missteps are unintentional, of course. Yet I still wonder whether an innocent lapse points to some confusion inherent in our nomenclature or in our understanding. "Medial lemniscus" isn't the "medial longitudinal fasciculus," for example. The median forebrain bundle isn't found only in the forebrain. A subtler error, still related to a problem with names, is a confusion between a/the "nucleus/i of the posterior commissure" (there are such nuclei) and, say, the interstitial nucleus of Cajal and the nucleus of Darkschewitsch, both of whose fibers project into posterior commissure. Is a phenomenon like Collier's sign, mentioned at the end of the last chapter, the result of a nuclear lesion or of a white-matter disconnection of some type? One last example among so many accrued over years: "it's a colliculus, but one can't tell whether it's the superior one or the inferior one." Wrong. One can. The superior one is laminated; the inferior one isn't.

Let's state the obvious for the record: nobody at any school or anywhere else seeks embarrassment by way of their misstatements, but they're universal and common—both the misstatements and the embarrassment. A cover-up that often ensues is usually far worse than the error was in the first place.

It's all perfectly OK; we're just trying to learn.

*

All the same, as I think about an axial section of midbrain below the level of the central caudal nucleus, I see in front of my eyes the bright, beacon-like, neatly round, small, midline-hugging CN IV nuclei. They stare at me, and they're all the more obvious when the section is stained such that white matter is black. Blackness of white matter in a Weil or Loyez stain makes CN IV nuclei even more obvious in their intimate relationship to the very dark medial longitudinal fasciculus (MLF), in which the nuclei are nestled–"sunken" is another description. We know that MLF exists above the level of CN III nuclear complex, and we'll see how it extends well below CN VI nuclei in the pons.

Assuming that one doesn't have a demonic axial section that cuts very obliquely, the colliculus at the level of CN IV nuclei is inferior, not superior.

We apply our principle related to the cerebral aqueduct in midbrain and rostral pons. Per **RULE #5** (from chapter 5: find the cerebral aqueduct; if you don't find it, you're not in midbrain), it's there, surrounded by periaqueductal grey, so midbrain is a reasonable, albeit not exclusive possibility regarding our location (remember, cerebral aqueduct is also present in the high pons).

Now we divide and organize.

DORSAL/ALAR/SENSORY NUCLEI. We'll concentrate on **inferior colliculus**, the conspicuous sensory nucleus in our current field of view. Yet we should re-acknowledge the presence, at this level as in the last, of the mesencephalic nucleus of CN V in the lateral borders of the periaqueductal grey on either side.

*

In a draft of this short section, I followed the approach of textbooks: I described the auditory pathway, but with emphasis on how the inferior colliculus contributes to an "attention to sound" rather than to physical characteristics like sound frequency, intensity, interaural time differences between either ear, etc. (Ono and Ito, 1985).

I like the phrase "attention to sound." It evokes a sense of Nauta's head turn towards an unseen target as a function of superior colliculus, discussed previously. Both the superior and inferior colliculi are somewhat mis-described as being visual and auditory, respectively, because there are ways in which both structures must be multimodal.

I scrapped my draft, because this monograph isn't a textbook and doesn't pretend to be. It's a discussion of one person's approach to the brainstem. Regarding inferior colliculus, I have an idiosyncratic view of it. So, here's a vignette and digression.

I use my 128-hertz tuning fork everyday to test patients' vibratory sense (the lemniscal pathway). I strike the fork; I apply it to the great toe. Over the years, I've come to tap the fork ever so lightly. In medical school, I banged it like *Homo habilis* using an early tool. Then as now, obviously, I'm producing sound waves of different intensities, but my intention with my 128-hertz instrument at someone's foot is to test a system that starts with a mechanoreceptor in soft tissue, not to test hearing. The sensory pathway I test shares the word "lemniscus" with a structure in the auditory pathway. (The *medial* lemniscus relates to how vibratory information finds its way to somatosensory thalamus; the *lateral* lemniscus has to do with the auditory pathway. A "lemniscus" is a "ribbon"-like structure, and indeed both medial and lateral lemnisci ribbon-wind their way rostrally.)

It should come as no surprise that the **lateral lemniscus** is present in our current axial section; its white matter seems part of the inferior colliculi. The lateral lemniscus is dorsal to both the medial lemniscus and the spinothalamic tract. The lateral lemniscus *differs* from yet another tract that's also quite lateral in midbrain, the **brachium of inferior colliculus**. The latter is lateral to *both* the inferior and superior colliculi in consecutive axial sections. The brachium of inferior colliculus connects inferior colliculus to medial geniculate body of thalamus. It's not a direct continuation of lateral lemniscus.

Memories have a peculiar way of sticking together. When I used to bang at my turning fork, my patients regularly said, "yes, I hear that."

How could they not? Then, in a separate but related memory, for years upon years, I watched colleagues and students point in the general area of the lateral, dorsal midbrain, and they'd say "there's medial lemniscus, or brachium of inferior colliculus, or lateral lemniscus, or spinothalamic tract. *They're all there.*" Those persons weren't incorrect; but it all seemed hand-wavingly vague to me. But my glued-together memories have left me with a notion that there must be relationship between auditory and tactile vibrations.

Enter the interesting question (to me) of whether snakes—boas, rattlesnakes, what have you—*hear*, or whether they primarily sense ground vibration. As it happens, the structures of the snake jaw—a "columella" akin to stapes; a "quadrate" akin to incus; and the snake mandible, which contacts the ground as malleus contacts the tympanic membrane—serve as inner-ear ossicles. And, just to let you know, snakes have eighth cranial nerves.

The supposedly earless snake "hears" both by sound and by ground vibration, and *both data sets project onto a snake's version of the inferior colliculus* (Hartline, 1971). I think about that observation whenever I see inferior colliculus, and—I whisper this next part to myself—maybe there's a reason for the anatomical proximity of a facial proprioceptive center (mesencephalic nucleus of CN V, related to the jaw, no less) and the fiber tracts of the medial and lateral lemnisci.

*

VENTRAL/BASAL/MOTOR NUCLEI. Here's an official-sounding description of **CN IV nucleus**: "The trochlear nucleus (IV) lies in the midbrain ventral to the aquaeduct [sic]. In humans, it has been observed to consist of one large [motor neuron or 'motoneuron'] group 'sunken' into the MLF; and several smaller groups of motoneurons further caudally. . ... It contains only motoneurons of the contralateral superior oblique [SO] muscle; however the contribution of SO motor unit activity during some types of eye movements such as convergence . . . is still not well understood" (Büttner-Ennever, 2006). I quote the passage for two reasons.

The first has to do with an idea, mentioned at the start of the last chapter and the beginning of this one, that CN IV nucleus represents a caudal appendage of CN III nuclear complex. If little motoneuron collections extend further caudally from the more-obvious, central bulk of CN IV nucleus, then couldn't we start to envision a very medially located "column" of somatic motoneurons beginning in midbrain?

One approach to brainstem has been to organize it into functional units that span the rostral-caudal axis, though "the classical division of the brainstem into *functional columns* has been a problem because it has proved difficult to delimit terms . . ." (my italics, Müller and O'Rahilly, 2011). I agree: terms like "special" vs. "general" "visceral" efferent don't help me as much as they might other people. We'll address columns in chapters 8, 10, and when we arrive in medulla.

Second, the author doesn't say that CN IV nucleus *uniquely* innervates a contralateral muscle, because we know of other subnuclei that involve either complete or partial decussation to their respective muscles—e.g., the superior rectus subnucleus or the central caudal nucleus, as discussed in the last chapter.

Nevertheless, since CN IV motoneurons innervate contralateral superior oblique motor units, then the infranuclear fascicle or the nerve itself must cross the midline. The former claim about the fascicle, not the latter about the extra-axial nerve, is true: "Root [fascicular] fibers emerging from the [CN IV] nucleus curve dorsolaterally and caudally in the outer margin of the central [periaqueductal] gray, decussate completely in the superior medullary velum and exit from the dorsal surface of the brain stem caudal to the inferior colliculus" (Carpenter and Sutin, 1983).

*

We've concentrated on CN IV nuclei, but we should re-acknowledge the white matter tracts we've previously encountered:

> **central tegmental tract** (a still-visible portion of the reticular formation, lateral to a centrally located

decussation of the superior cerebellar peduncles; the red nuclei are no longer visible, because we are below them), and, laterally, the **spinothalamic and medial lemniscal tracts**.

We're not done with **VENTRAL/MOTOR NUCLEI** aside from CN IV nuclei. But on the subject of white matter tracts ventral to the inferior colliculi, one must ask, with amazement, if not incredulity: *why all the white-matter midline crossings at our present axial level?*

In the 1940's, an anatomist wondered whether the trochlear decussation had to do with the embryonic appearance of the cerebellum (Cooper, 1947). At the level of the inferior colliculi, the dominant decussation we see is that of the superior cerebellar peduncles (in an appropriately stained section, it's a big blob of black inside the midline tegmentum, dorsal to the cerebral peduncles), but there are other crossings worth considering. At the isthmus between lower midbrain and the remaining hindbrain a number of "transactions" appear before us in a limited anatomic space:

> deep cerebellar nuclear axons (they ascend) cross to the contralateral red nuclei (as mentioned, via the **decussation of the superior cerebellar peduncles** or brachia conjunctivae);
>
> tectum (particularly, the superior colliculus) projects to spinal cord (the projections descend and cross in the **dorsal tegmental decussation**, which is also known as **the fountain decussation of Meynert**);
>
> tectum projects to mesencephalic reticular formation (bilaterally) and to contralateral pontine and medullary reticular formation (also via the dorsal tegmental decussation);
>
> and red nucleus projects either to contralateral spinal cord (the projections descend and cross in the **ventral tegmental decussation**), or they project to ipsilateral

medulla, without decussation, via the **central tegmental tract** (Nathan and Smith, 1982).

So, at the level of the trochlear decussation and the decussation of the superior cerebellar peduncles, we pivot to the bridge that is pons:

> The decussation of the trochlear nerve in the superior medullary velum and the rostral edge of the pons mark the border of the mesencephalon [read: midbrain] and the metencephalon [read: pons] on the dorsal and ventral sides of the brainstem, respectively, and the decussation of the superior cerebellar peduncle marks the transition of the tegmentum pontis into the tegmentum mescenphali (Nieuwenhuys et al., 2008).

In some sections of low midbrain, you visualize the transition from cerebral peduncles to the tegmentum pontis. And in that ventral domain are **VENTRAL/MOTOR NUCLEI** in abundance, specifically the pontine nuclei, about which more when we get to pons.

*

> **RULE #6**. The person who says "it's not important clinically" could be horribly mistaken.

RULE #6 is just an opinion based on thousands of hours watching how we teach students. Out of necessity, we choose certain things to emphasize–that's both proper and practical. But throwing out too many details is like dismissing pertinent positives in talking with patients. The consequences of doing so can be less than delightful.

So, what's a person to do? One can't commit everything to memory.

Here's an approach that I've found useful, if time consuming. Based on curiosity alone, ask "what *is* that?" Then, if you're so inclined, you spend hours ferreting out your answer. I have two examples in mind, as we prepare to depart from midbrain to pons.

Example 1: the periaqueductal (or central) grey. It's grey or (if you prefer the occidental spelling) "gray," right? So, it must consist of neurons, but are they divisible into dorsal/sensory and ventral/motor populations? We admitted from the start that our alar/basal dividing line in midbrain and rostral pons is an oversimplification. Moreno-Bravo et al. (2012) note that genetic differentiation to distinguish alar or basal plate neuronal origin in the periaqueductal grey is less well characterized than elsewhere in the midbrain, but they also note that although there are neurons there, they don't obviously collect into nuclei.

But we continue to ask: what *is* it? Nauta and Feirtag (1986) teach about the periaqueductal grey effortlessly; the italics are mine:

> The central gray substance has long been known as a destination for fibers that travel with the spinothalamic tract *but do not attain the thalamus*. It also receives projections from cerebral cortex, the hypothalamus, and the reticular formation. Its outputs are no less heterogeneous: it projects upward to the hypothalamus and the superior colliculus, *radially outward to the surrounding reticular formation, and downward to the rhombencephalic reticular formation*, the nucleus of the solitary tract, and the dorsal motor nucleus of the vagus.

The only part of the surrounding mesencephalic reticular formation that we've visualized is the central tegmental tract, which passes from red nucleus to caudal points (it also contains fibers which ascend to cortex). But there's a larger network/reticulum that we don't see, though it's invisibly present, as someone once described *"the* nothing that is," throughout the brainstem.

Example 2: *I'll withhold the name for a moment.* Between exiting fascicles of both oculomotor nerves, in the very ventral tegmentum, *immediately* dorsal to the interpeduncular fossa, is a midline, solitary nucleus that's close to the ventral tegmental area of Tsai. It has pigmented cells in it. What *is* that?

Trust me: the more you ask the question sincerely, the more you learn. For a discussion of the connectivities we open up by introducing this structure, see Hikosaka, 2010.

It's name describes its location: the **interpeduncular nucleus**, which is highly conserved across vertebrate species. It communicates with epithalamus via **fasciculus retroflexus** or the **habenula-interpeduncular tract**, whose medially placed fibers contribute to what seems like a white-matter capsule surrounding the red nuclei on either side. Recall that we started at the interface between epithalamus and mesencephalon. Here, as we leave midbrain, there's a structure in bent-back communication with rostral epithalamus. It's not a somatic motor nucleus; it *is* of basal plate origin; it receives from the habenulae, and it projects to midline nuclei in the "raphe," a "seam" or "suture" (from the Greek) best seen in pons.

7.

Rostral Pons

The look of the cerebral aqueduct has changed. In midbrain, it's more or less a circle. At the transition to the pons, I'd say that it looks quadrilateral. The dorsal two edges, which meet in the midline to form an inverted "V", form the thin roof which we identified in the previous chapter as the **superior medullary velum**. Infranuclear fascicles from CN IV nuclei decussate through it. (Depending on the brain you're studying, the circular aqueduct could also change its appearance to something more like a "Y" shape; the point's still the same: it's look has changed.) We're at the rostral extent of the fourth ventricle, but atlases still refer to the cerebral aqueduct's presence in the high pons.

Applying the principle that **DORSAL/ALAR/SENSORY NUCLEI** lie above the aqueduct, we find mesencephalic nucleus of CN V on either side of the aqueduct, dorsal to a bluish nucleus which appears at this level.

The superior medullary velum is of alar-plate origin as the cerebellum is of alar-plate origin. So, one can't say that alar structures have vanished; rather, the superior medullary velum is a first suggestion of cerebellum (Müller and O'Rahilly, 1988). As an aside, both the pons and the cerebellar hemispheres in humans are inordinately large compared to all other species.

Superior, middle, and inferior cerebellar peduncles—the three white-matter struts which connect brainstem to cerebellum and vice versa—will serve as landmarks for the remainder of our tour.

*

To clarify terms, there are people who refer to the dorsal/upper half of the pons at this level as the **pontine tegmentum**, whereas the ventral/lower/larger portion goes by names like "the pons proper" or the **basis pontis**. (Note the difference, compared to midbrain: tectum is dorsal and tegmentum is ventral.) There's still a roof (tectum) in the rostral pons, however: the **superior medullary velum**, and, more caudally, the **inferior medullary velum** cover the fourth ventricle, which widens as we pass lower into the pons, are both alar and tectal. Structures like the superior cerebellar peduncle, the extensive white matter of the middle cerebellar peduncle, the inferior cerebellar peduncle, and cerebellum itself will also dorsally tent the fourth ventricle. More on all those structures in time.

The 16th century Italian anatomist, Constanzo Varolio, who first assigned the term "pons" to pons, thought that it was a bridge (Italian, *ponte*; French, *pont*; Latin, *pons*) between cerebellar hemispheres. His 1573 book contains a curious illustration in which he split the brainstem lengthwise while it's still attached to the brain, then he splayed the brainstem's two lengthwise halves in different directions; he had to have cut the dorsal midline cerebellum to accomplish this perspective (Bahsi et al., 2018). Varolio thought that pons was a passage from side to side, not from hemispheres to hindbrain.

In axial section, the basis pontis to me looks symmetrical from side to side just as the midbrain does, but instead of ventral cerebral peduncles, we have the appearance of a slightly cleft chin (a large one, a bit bilobed) with a midline seam or suture that passes from the ventral surface all the way to the cerebral aqueduct. If you visualize the great amount of white matter in the basis pontis, some fibers seem pass from side to side and others pass from above to below.

In the tegmentum ventral to the aqueduct, we re-acknowledge the white matter tracts we've previously encountered:

> **medial longitudinal fasciculus** at the midline, ventral to aqueduct;
>
> **tectospinal tract**, which has arisen from superior colliculus and whose fibers have crossed in the **dorsal tegmental decussation**; tectospinal tract is just ventral to the medial longitudinal fasciculus and remains intimately proximate to it throughout brainstem;
>
> **superior cerebellar peduncles**, which occupy much of the tegmentum at this level, on either side; they have not decussated at this level (we're lower, compared to last chapter);
>
> **central tegmental tract**, whose white matter seems to blend into superior cerebellar peduncle on the latter's medial side;
>
> **spinothalamic and medial lemniscal tracts**, ventral to **superior cerebellar peduncle**;
>
> and, dorsolaterally, **lateral lemniscus**.

VENTRAL/BASAL NUCLEI. I'll quote Nauta and Feirtag (1986) once more, this time on the subject of the bluish nucleus mentioned a moment ago; the italics, again, are mine:

> The transmitter norepinephrine is employed by the *locus ceruleus*, a group of roughly 20,000 neurons extending from *the ventrolateral corner of the central gray substance some distance into the adjacent tegmentum* . . .. The region indeed is cerulean, or distinctly dark blue in color, both in fresh brains and in brains fixed in formaldehyde. The blueness reflects the region's content of neuromelanin, a pigment synthesized by most of the neurons of the locus. The pigment is a polymer of dihydroxyphenylalanine, or DOPA, the precursor of

the catecholamine neurotransmitters. Apart from its chemical properties, the locus ceruleus is remarkable anatomically: its *efferents are distributed to all the main divisions of the central nervous system*. On average, then, its 20,000 neurons must each influence a very great number of neurons elsewhere in the brain. In that respect, *the locus ceruleus is a caricature of the reticular formation: it embodies the extreme expression of a prominent reticular trait, an apparent diffuseness and nonspecificity of synaptic connections.*

As in their discussion of central or periaqueductal grey, they allude to an aspect of brainstem anatomy that doesn't lend itself to a point-at-a-thing-and-name-it approach. *Diffuseness and nonspecificity of synaptic connections*: it's a concept worth elaborating now.

Certainly you can point to **locus ceruleus** in a gross specimen. As plain to the eye as that nucleus is, a largely unseen network–which calls to mind Camille Golgi's notion of branching arborization as a key to microanatomy (his "reticularism," as opposed to Ramon y Cajal's "neuronism" [Jones, 1999 and Sterling, 1998])–is present throughout brainstem. We're not just talking about the reticular formation, whether mesencephalic or rhombencephalic. We also refer to a number of diffuse systems and their arbors.

Let's discuss three of them, all represented in the rostral pons.

We teach that locus cerulean neurons synthesize norepinephrine. We say that **nuclei of the raphe**–the raphe being the seam or suture mentioned earlier–synthesize serotonin, an indolamine. We refer to a cholinergic zone (it seems to me more a zone than a nucleus; there are cholinergic neurons even in the central grey) in the lateral tegmentum of the high pons. A cholinergic **pedunculopontine nucleus** has been of interest in the modern treatment of Parkinson's disease, because long-term stimulation of the area may improve gait (Aravamuthan et al., 2007). All the anatomic-structural associations mentioned– locus ceruleus with norepinephrine, raphe nuclei with serotonin, and pedunculopotine nucleus with acetylcholine–are essentially correct, but they are simplifications compared to the true anatomy.

The locus ceruleus accounts for perhaps only 50% of neurons that synthesize norepinephrine; the remainder of catecholaminergic neurons are found in less discretely bounded locales through the pontine and medullary tegmentum. Whereas serotonergic neurons can be found in multiple nuclei the hug the midline raphe, not all raphe nuclear neurons are serotonergic; indeed, probably only a minority of neurons in many raphe nuclei are indolaminergic. Finally, cholinergic neurons don't occupy a neat grey unit either; they seem instead to be scattered not only in the area of pedunculopontine nucleus, but also in the so-called **medial and lateral parabrachial nuclei of rostral pons**.

We teach about projections from the above nuclei or zones to diverse locales–*efferents distributed to all the main divisions of the central nervous system*, per Nauta and Feirtag. Consider cholinergic axons:

> Cholinergic neurons . . . in the mesopontine reticular formation (particularly the pedunculopontine nucleus) compose the major excitatory reticulothalamic pathway to the nonspecific thalamocortical system; they influence this system by direct excitation of thalamocortical neurons, as well as by disinhibition of the thalamic reticular nucleus (Kinney and Samuels, 1994).

Studious attempts have been made to follow cholinergic projections to thalamus and elsewhere, but one wonders whether one loses a sense of "the tree" by obsessive attention to branches.

That said, here are some basics regarding neurotransmitter projections from dispersed, high pontine locales:

> Many, not all, cholinergic projections ascend in the **dorsal tegmental pathway**, also known as the **dorsal longitudinal fasciculus** (Shute and Lewis, 1967).

Many, not all, noradrenergic fibers ascend via the **central tegmental tract** and **median forebrain bundle** to cortical destinations (Nieuwenhuys, 1985).

Some, not all, serotonergic fibers pass via **dorsal tegmental pathway** and **median forebrain bundle** to rostral points (Nieuwenhuys, 1985).

The pathways mentioned are typically bidirectional. So, hypothalamic axons also descend in the **dorsal tegmental pathway**, although there's debate over whether, for example, projections from parvocululuar paraventricular nucleus of hypothalamus connect monosynaptically with neurons in the spinal cord's intermediolateral grey column, from whence second-order arise in the sympathetic pupillodilatory pathway (Carpenter and Sutin, 1983 and Burnstock, 2009).

VENTRAL/MOTOR NUCLEI. There are theories, but no one really knows what cortical information transmits via the **frontopontine** and **temporopontine tracts**—the bundles of Arnold and Türck, respectively—to **pontine nuclei**. Nor is it trivial to map those nuclei. There are clever people who have imported neuroimages of pontine infarctions into a Photoshop program to create topographies (maps) of rostral/basal motor fibers and nuclei, based on associated clinical deficits:

> The syndromes are not absolutely discrete . . ..
> Structure-function correlations indicate that strength is conveyed by the corticofugal fibers destined for spinal cord, whereas dysmetria results from lesions involving the neurons of the basilar pons [basis pontis] that link the ipsilateral cerebral cortex with the contralateral cerebellar hemisphere (Schmahmann et al., 2004).

To quibble momentarily, the word "corticofugal" (*fugere*, Latin, to flee) needs some qualification. It's not that homolateral cortico-pontine fibers heading to contralateral cerebellar hemisphere, via pontine connections, aren't also "fleeing" cortex. They do. The authors want to distinguish between how damage to a certain population of fibers can result *in weakness* as opposed to how pontine-nuclear damage or a lesion of pontocerebellar fibers can result in *incoordination* that's disproportionate to whatever weakness there may be, if any. The distinction can be hard to judge, given the physical proximity of *both* corticofugal systems in the pons.

There are generalizations we can consider, based on the authors' correlations. In the rostral pons, facial strength is represented dorsomedially; articulation (the *coordination* of movements to produce speech) is ventromedial. Swallowing maps all through rostral pons, medially, laterally, and ventrally. In a very overlapping way, hand and arm strength and coordination map to ventral basis pontis. We describe just the rostral pons for the time being.

*

Pontine nuclei: what *are* they? Based on studies in cats, two provocative theorists (Blomfield and Marr, 1970) talk about the one thing that they can confidently say about cortico-cerebellar intercommunication. By way of serial monosynaptic connections, it's fast:

> . . . discharges in the pontine nuclei follow stimulation of the cerebral white matter by as little as 2 ms [milliseconds]. . . . Contextual information reaching the cerebellar cortex through the mossy fibres is also rapidly transmitted . . . . The time taken for stimulation of the subcortical white matter to evoke a mossy fibre response is 2.7 ms.

If you're curious about other conduction in an informational loop that returns from cerebellum to cortex, the intervals are also speedy:

> . . . pontine nuclei to cerebellar nuclei, 1 ms [this projection exists, perhaps, to our surprise]; cerebellar

nuclei to VL [ventrolateral] nucleus of thalamus, 2 ms; VL nucleus of thalamus to [layer V or "Betz"] cerebral pyramidal cells, an estimated 1 ms.

The role of pontine nuclei seems more than the transfer of action potentials across the midline to contralateral cerebellum; projections from those nuclei to deep cerebellar nuclei hint at a positive feedback loop in which ". . . a movement–once initiated–will tend to continue indefinitely (at least well beyond the normal firing period of pyramidal cells in response to excitatory input): and this will only be terminated either by applying direct inhibition to the deep pyramidal cells or by breaking the feedback loop."

That the theory is old shouldn't worry us. It's of use to illustrate that pontine nuclei may be involved in moment-to-moment motor control. They aren't merely internuncial or "connector" neurons.

8.

Properly in the Fourth Ventricle

Where the cerebral aqueduct once was in previous axial sections, now we visualize a widening quadrilateral space, which is the fourth ventricle. I imagine myself inside that ventricle, and I want to know what's above, below, and to the sides of me.

Don't forget **RULE #4**. We apply the following to all our axial sections: ventral brainstem is *below* dorsal brainstem. (In MR and CT images, unlike anatomic sections, ventral brainstem is above dorsal brainstem.)

I stand astride the midline suture or median sulcus that divides symmetrical halves of the pons; my feet are on the floor of the fourth ventricle. On either side of the midline (my feet barely apart), my feet touch the so-called median eminences, in modern anatomical parlance. But anatomists of a former time referred to "round bundles," which are the **medial longitudinal fasciculi** inside the eminences. If I reach up to touch the fastigium (top) above me, my fingers touch the under side of the **superior medullary velum**, but dorsal to that velum is the most rostral–and rather tiny–lobule of the cerebellar vermis, the **lingula**.

I seem to be under a kind of gambrel roof; to either side of my outstretched arms, the margins are at acute angles to the fourth ventricular floor. The superior cerebellar peduncles tent me dorsolaterally.

These superior peduncles go by another name, the brachia conjunctivae (singular: **brachium conjunctivum**).

A brachium is an arm. The Latin root of conjunctivum is a verb having to do with joining or connection. For example, the conjunctivum *of the eye* conjoins the eyeball surface to that of the inner eyelid. So, what does a brachium conjunctivum connect? In the 19th century, there was a thought about a bending commissure between deep cerebellar nuclei on one side and the inferior olive on the other (Voogd and van Baarsen, 2014). That's not the modern view, but it's interesting. Keep in mind that the central tegmental tract is very close to the tegmental brachium conjunctivum before the latter decussates. The **central tegmental tract** is a boulevard traversed by fibers from red nucleus to homolateral inferior olive. Add the contralateral **den-tate nucleus** of cerebellum and you've identified the vertices of a **rubro-olivary-dentate triangle (of Guillain and Mollaret**), lesions of which are associated with certain tremors or myoclonus.[1]

The oddity and interest of the superior cerebellar peduncle is its *dorsolateral* presence at the roof of the fourth ventricle, its *ventromedial* location in rostral pontine tegmentum, and thence to what we've called (in an appropriately stained section) a "big blob of black" in the midbrain tegmentum, i.e., the **decussation of superior cerebellar**

---

[1] If (left) red nucleus, (left) inferior olive, and (right) dentate nucleus are the vertices, what are the sides of the triangle of Guillain and Mollaret? (Left) red nucleus and (left) inferior olive connect via the central tegmental tract without fibers crossing the midline. (Right) dentate projects to (left) red nucleus via the superior cerebellar peduncle. There is a medullary olivocerebellar projection: (left) olivary fibers cross the midline in medulla to project to contralateral (right) dentate via the (right) inferior cerebellar peduncle (Ruigrok TJH and Voogd J, 2000), although there's controversy about whether the last of the three sides is relevant to the pathology of palatal myoclonus (Lapresle and Hamida, 1970).

It's been further observed that palatal myoclonus associated with lesions of the triangle is side-specific: myoclonus occurs on the side opposite lesions of the olive and central tegmental tract, but on the same side in cerebellar lesions (Gautier and Blackwood, 1961). From that 1961 paper (cases 2 and 3), "twitching of the palate" towards the right was associated with left inferior olivary changes in both, but right dentate pathology in case 2 and left central tegmental tract pathology in case 3.

peduncles. The superior cerebellar peduncle is the largest efferent tract leaving cerebellum; it's an arm that bends in space to reach across the midline. Its axons (say, in the right brachium conjunctivum) arise from (right) dentate nucleus, the most lateral of the (right) deep cerebellar nuclei. The (right) superior cerebellar peduncle connects (right) deep cerebellar nuclei with red nucleus and, mainly, with thalamus on the contralateral (left) side.

Looking up at the dorsolateral roof of the fourth ventricle, I have no presentiment that the brachium conjunctivum will cross the midline: all I know is that the left brachium has arisen from left cerebellum, right brachium from right cerebellum. I'd have to track an axon in one peduncle along its entire course to convince myself that there's a crossing. In the eyes of Galen of Greek antiquity, the brachium conjunctivum simply looked like a "tendon" of brain; he didn't observe its decussating path (Voogd and van Baarsen, 2014). At the present level, one appreciates the early Greek observation.

*

I'm still standing inside the fourth ventricle. Gazing again at its floor, assuming that my view isn't obscured by choroid plexus or a lattice of vessels, I'm interested in the lateral edge, at the acutest angle formed by the floor and the slant gable of superior cerebellar peduncle above it. Neurosurgical colleagues would say that there's no obvious landmark there, certainly not as plain as the so-called facial colliculi on the fourth ventricular floor at a level caudal to where we are now. Anatomy colleagues might say that the **sulcus limitans** (described by Wilhelm His, Sr. in the 19th century; his son, the junior, described the bundle of His in the heart) isn't as clearly present anatomically here as it is, for example, in medulla.

Is it possible to distinguish alar from basal nuclei at our current level? Keep in mind that, in development, neurons might originate in basal plate, but they translocate to lateral positions by maturity (Puelles et al., 2018). Yet, at the very lateral corner of the fourth ventricle, here at the level of the **principal sensory and motor nuclei of CN V** (which are deep and lateral to the corner), the principal sensory nucleus *is dorsolateral* to the principle motor nucleus. There's also a bit of the **mesencephalic trigeminal nucleus** at the current level: applying the simplification that sensory nuclei are lateral to motor ones, we'd surmise that mesencephalic trigeminal nucleus is lateral to the principal motor nucleus—which it is.

In short, division into alar/dorsal/lateral (= sensory) and basal/ventral/medial (= motor) might not be perfect, but it's a serviceable way of thinking about important brainstem nuclei. Note that the distinction we mentioned in midbrain—a division between alar/dorsal/sensory nuclei and basal/ventral/motor nuclei—tilts its axis such that sensory nuclei are now *lateral* to motor nuclei.

Nieuwenhuys (2011) has strong views on the subject:

> According to His (1891, 1893) the brainstem consists of two longitudinal zones, the dorsal alar plate (sensory in nature) and the ventral basal plate (motor in nature). [John Black] Johnston and [C. Judson] Herrick [both Americans, who published in the very early 20th century] indicated that both plates can be subdivided into separate somatic and visceral zones, distinguishing somatosensory and viscerosensory zones with the alar plate, and visceromotor and somatomotor zones within the basal plate. . . . Recent developmental molecular studies on brains of birds and mammals confirmed the presence of longitudinal zones, and also showed molecularly defined transverse bands or neuromeres throughout development . . .. [I]t may be hypothesized that the brainstems of all vertebrates share a basic organizational plan, in which intersecting longitudinal and transverse zones form fundamental histogenetic and genoarchitectonic units.

All I want to do is keep organizing my anatomical information. At our current pontine level, the mesencephalic and principal sensory nuclei of CN V are lateral to the principal motor nucleus in the tegmentum.

Elsewhere in that tegmentum, ventral to the floor of fourth ventricle, we re-acknowledge the white matter tracts we've previously encountered:

> **medial longitudinal fasciculus** at the midline, below my feet;
> **tectospinal tract**, just below the medial longitudinal fasciculus, retaining its intimate proximity to it;
> **central tegmental tract**, which is less obvious than in higher sections;
> **spinothalamic and medial lemniscal tracts**, ventral to the central tegmental tract;
> and, dorsolaterally, **lateral lemniscus**;
> the **pyramidal tracts** appear to be condensing into a discrete white-matter bundles in the ventral basis pontis.

VENTRAL/MOTOR PONTINE NUCLEI. Recall our Photoshop colleagues from chapter 7; we cite them again (Schmahmann et al., 2004). In the pons at the level of CN V nuclei, facial strength isn't much represented; neither is articulation. Instead, strength maps to ventral basis pontis (where the pyramidal tract is, now more obviously than in more superior sections). Coordination of a leg maps to presumptive pontine nuclei located in dorsal and dorsolateral basis pontis; coordination of gait maps, frankly, all over the place: to the most ventral basis pontis at our previous (higher) level, our current one, and also caudal to our present level.

*

Regarding the conspicuous appearance of the **middle cerebellar peduncle**, to either side of the pons laterally, let's distill information about it:

a. It's also called the **brachium pontis**.

In axial section, one doesn't quite appreciate the sweeping course of the brachia.

Warning, here comes a gratuitous association. I think about a statue in the Louvre in Paris, from the Hellenistic period, named the Winged Victory of Samothrace. It's striking. Nine feet tall. It's a headless and armless woman, draped in flowing garments that draft against her body and behind her, as if in an oncoming wind. She has immense wings which extend behind her. If you stand directly in front of her (you gaze up, because she stands on a pedestal), the leading edge of the wings seem level with the shoulders; the wing feathers dangle down. In that one view of her outspread wings, I visualize the sweeping course of the medial cerebellar peduncles on either side of the pons.

b. The middle cerebellar peduncle is the largest afferent pathway into cerebellum, "quantitatively the most important route by which the cerebral cortex can influence cerebellar cortex" (Carpenter and Sutin, 1983). Projections from much of cortex (frontal motor, dorsolateral prefrontal, parietal, and superior temporal—at least those locales) descend to pontine nuclei on the same side, then second-order axons in the middle cerebellar peduncle decussate into the medullary core of the contralateral cerebellar hemisphere.

c. In the pontine tegmentum, transversely oriented fibers that will make up the middle cerebellar peduncles pass both dorsal and ventral to the descending fibers of the pyramidal tract. The anatomic proximity of structures related to coordination and to strength makes one think that, here, ataxia and hemiparesis could simultaneously result from a discrete lesion. Nevertheless, regarding the case we discussed in our chapter 2, a curious point arises: ". . . it is not clear why the cerebellar signs are not bilateral" (Fisher, 1978). What passes from left to right also passes from right to left, hence the question of why a unilateral lesion wouldn't result in bilateral signs.

9.

Beyond Brazis

If you've forgotten who Brazis is (admittedly, chapter 2 was a long time ago), he's the author of chapter 14 of *Localization in Clinical Neurology*. I return to him and to the case discussed in our chapter 2 now that we're half-way into our tour of axial brainstem sections. It's a reasonable moment to take stock of where we've been.

Here is Brazis's summary of an ataxic hemiparesis:

> ATAXIC HEMIPARESIS. A lesion (usually a lacunar infarction) in the basis pontis at the junction of the upper one-third and lower two-thirds of the pons may result in the ataxic-hemiparesis (homolateral ataxia and crural [related to the leg] paresis) syndrome. In this syndrome hemiparesis, which is more severe in the lower extremity, is associated with ipsilateral hemiataxia and occasionally dysarthria, nystagmus, and paresthesias. The lesion is in the contralateral pons. This syndrome has also been has also been described with contralateral thalamocapsular lesions (Brazis, 1985).

Eighty-three words in length, the description is not only mercifully short, but also it repeats itself, I assume, for emphasis: "ataxic hemiparesis" is mentioned twice; then we have "homolateral ataxia and *crural* paresis" followed by an iterative description ("hemiparesis, *which is more severe in the lower extremity*, . . . associated with ipsilateral hemiataxia . . ."). We learn two possible localizations, both textbook. The one in brainstem is rather precise, "at the junction of the upper one-third and lower two-thirds of the pons"–which is about the location where we ended the preceding chapter. I take the paragraph to be of the tell-them-what-you-are-going-to-say-then-say-it-then-tell-them-what-you-just-said school of instruction.

Yet if I confidently talk about a left pontine localization for a right-sided ataxic hemiparesis, because Brazis echoes in my head, then I tacitly violate **RULES #1** and **#2**.

The 44 year-old man in our second chapter had no dysarthria, but a left-beating nystagmus, diminished optokinetic nystagmus (OKN) with leftward moving targets, and a sense that the right hand (only) was swollen or stiff, in the absence of a sensory deficit. Most of all, he had a motor problem that invites one "to postulate a single site along the cerebral neuraxis where pyramidal and cerebellar signs would not be contralateral to each other" (Fisher, 1978).

The authors whom I've affectionately called Photoshop colleagues (the lead author works across town) teach me the following, based on studies in monkeys:

> . . . pontocerebellar fibres from one side of the pons traverse the opposite hemipons, and disperse amongst numerous, widely divergent pontocerebellar fascicles before coalescing into the opposite brachium pontis. Together with the motor corticopontine projections that terminate in multiple discrete regions in the middle and caudal pons, this arrangement may account for the absence of ipsilateral dysmetria in all but the largest infarcts. In smaller lesions, sufficient numbers of pontocerebellar fibres from the intact hemipons escape damage as they bypass the lesion on their way to the cerebellum, thus preventing ipsilateral dysmetria (Schmahmann et al., 2004).

OK, but does nystagmus and a paresthetic sense of swollen-ness (in just the right hand) make one think of a larger area of ischemia? Likewise, why did the man have such a problem *with his right arm*—recall that he couldn't light his cigarette; and, on finger-to-nose testing, wild oscillations caused him to strike his own face. Did an ischemic "penumbra" extend into higher pons? Is there anatomy that we haven't studied in enough depth to account for all the clinical findings, in the same way that we need to know about the ramification of pontocerebellar fibers before they coalesce in (contralateral) middle cerebellar peduncle to explain why the 44 year-old man's cerebellar findings aren't bilateral?

The OKN finding had me thinking at first about a right parietal (supratentorial) lesion; loss of OKN can happen in brainstem disease, but one might expect an accompanying gaze palsy (Davidoff et al., 1966). The unidirectional, leftward beating nystagmus had me thinking at first about a right vestibular problem, but unidirectional nystagmus could also be a dysfunction of gaze-holding mechanisms in brainstem (see chapter 10). The paresthetic right hand, if his sense of swelling or stiffness was a paresthesia, was significant to me simply because it was on the right side (I didn't know what to make of the sense, and he had no sensory deficit per se). All the above were lesser aspects of the presentation.

Regarding the ataxic hemiparesis itself (all its aspects, including falling to the right on Romberg testing), we repeat to ourselves that cerebellar and pyramidal tracts are closest to each other physically/anatomically in the midbrain or pons. Then we read how the original authors excluded the midbrain:

> If the responsible lesion were in the upper midbrain or subthalamic region it would be possible to involve the superior cerebellar peduncle after it has crossed the midline, and the cerebral peduncle lying immediately anterior to it, producing a combined cerebello-pyramidal disturbance on the opposite side. In our [case] . . . there were no signs of midbrain involvement such a third nerve palsy . . . (Fisher and Cole, 1965).

Why the right arm was so dyscoordinated still strikes me as curious. Perhaps the ischemia involved more rostral pons (where, perhaps, arm and hand are more generously represented, both in terms of strength and coordination), but, if so, one might have expected right arm weakness as well as bilateral cerebellar findings, given the larger affected territory.

We have no imaging or pathological correlation in the case.

*

To localize a lesion in left pons, at the junction of its upper one-third and lower two-thirds, is to invite consideration about how damage to certain structures rather than others disrupts what the brain is trying to accomplish in the first place.

Theorists talk about levels of analysis in trying to explain how the brain controls movement–the highest level relates to "the nature of the problem to be solved" (Alexander et al., 1994). In our patient's case, maybe the high-level problems included walking and lighting a cigarette. But certainly in this monograph, I'm at a very low level of analysis, and, yes, there's always anatomy that we can study in greater depth. Nor can we comment about whatever computations in different systems result in a normal gait or a lit cigarette. All that we seek is: to remain aware of distinct structures that are close to each other. Maybe we can start to understand principles of organization based on the anatomy's divisible proximities, such as that between principal sensory and motor nuclei of CN V or the non-overlapping nearness of cerebellar and pyramidal tracts in midbrain or pons.

10.

On the Facial Colliculus

June 17, 1858, a Thursday. A 43 year-old man, previously in good health except for a congenital atrophy of his right arm, had a restless night on the 16th. He didn't understand why he couldn't sleep. A bureaucrat of some type and apparently single, he earned enough money to satisfy his daily needs; he had a "penchant" for alcoholic beverages. He hadn't been ill recently. He recalled having a "brain fever" at age ten. In the early morning of the 17th, without cognizance of what had happened or how he got there, he was found down in the middle of a street. At first, he couldn't speak. He vomited copiously. By the time he got to hospital at 7 a.m., his mental state had cleared almost completely.

The first full examination we have dates to six days after his presentation. There were three findings: a right hemiparesis, a conjugate gaze paralysis looking to the left (both eyes couldn't look to the left in the horizontal plane), and a left facial paralysis–the last manifesting a smooth, unwrinked left forehead, an inability to close the left eyelids, and an effaced left nasolabial fold.

I'll cite the source later. For now, I want to keep the case in mind as we continue our tour of axial sections.

*

We're still in pons. I'm standing again in the fourth ventricle, and I want to know, yet again, what's above, below, and to the sides of me.

I stand astride the midline suture or median sulcus that divides symmetrical halves of the pons; my feet are on the floor of the fourth ventricle. But my footing is curious here. I feel that I stand on large domes on either side of the midline, and that the whole floor of the fourth is now more undulated than previously. My left foot balances on the left facial colliculus; my right on the right colliculus. So, what are these colliculi; why are they reliably identifiable landmarks in endoscopy of the fourth ventricle (Longetti et al., 2008); why do they exist in the first place? Another way of asking the last question is: why do facial-nerve fascicles on either side loop around CN VI (abducens) nuclei? Fascicular CN VII doesn't loop at all in the oldest branch of vertebrates represented by the lamprey (Pombal and Megías, 2018), and the "internal facial genu" in frogs and birds is nothing like what it is in humans (Fritzsch, 1998).

Here's a textbook answer:

> . . . the cell masses of the branchiomotor zone have migrated away from their original periventricular position. Their efferent fibers, however, have retained their original position. As a consequence, these fibers make a loop, directed at the floor of the fourth ventricle before they leave the brainstem in a lateral direction. In the case of the seventh nerve, this loop in known as the *genu* (knee) of the facial nerve. It can be recognized as an elevation in the floor of the fourth ventricle: the facial collicule [colliculus] (Nieuwenhuys et al., 2008).

Primordial facial branchiomotor neurons *move* from one place to another in development. They venture caudally to their mature location, inferior to CN VI nucleus (McKay et al., 1997), but I wonder whether "migration," whose path *is* the facial nerve's internal genu if you envision moving lateral to medial (though the efferent fibers pass medial to lateral), understates what we see in front of us.

We discuss a particularly complicated cranial nerve and its likewise complex functional circuitry (Chandrasekhar et al., 1997), since CN VII isn't only branchiomotor. It doesn't only innervate branchial arch-derived muscles that control facial expression. It's also secretomotor in its innervation of lacrimal and salivary glands, as well as sensory, in how it transmits afferent taste from the anterior two-thirds of the tongue as well as skin sensation from the ear's pinna and external auditory meatus. **Facial motor nucleus** (branchiomotor), **superior salivatory nucleus** (secretomotor), **nucleus of the solitary tract** (taste), and **spinal trigeminal nucleus** (sensation of outer ear) are responsible for their respective CN VII functions (Chandrasekhar, 2004). And if you follow the course of fascicular CN VII from its motor nucleus (caudal to CN VI nucleus) to the genu at the facial colliculus (where axons wrap around abducens nucleus at the facial collicule) to its exit at the pontomedullary junction, you find yourself at various points close to the discrete brainstem nuclei involved in all CN VII modalities.

*

Note to self: if there's a superior salivatory nucleus, there must be an inferior one, right? Not necessarily, as I read in Carpenter and Sutin (1983):

> [Superior salivatory nucleus is a] poorly defined nucleus . . .. Retrograde transport studies indicate that preganglionic parasympathetic neurons form an uninterrupted dorsal cell column extending from the medulla into the pons. Cells of the dorsal motor nucleus of the vagus form the more caudal portion of this column; cells in the more rostral regions are less compact and distributed over a wide region of the reticular formation. In the pons cells of this column lie between the nucleus of the solitary tract and the facial motor nucleus. The overlapping origins of neurons contributing to the glossopharyngeal [CN IX] and

intermediate nerve [that portion of CN VII carrying afferent sensory and efferent secretomotor fibers] raises a question concerning the appropriateness of a nomenclature that distinguishes separate salivatory nuclei as inferior and superior.

Is the above too much information for a monograph? No, and here's why: note the words "uninterrupted" and "cell column." Soon enough, we address more columns, what Nieuwenhuys (from chapter 8) calls longitudinal zones.

*

There's more to say about structures bounded within the dome of facial colliculus. The round bundle or medial longitudinal fasciculus still hugs the midline, as it did in our last, more rostral axial section. Then, there's the simply non-trivial matter of **CN VI (abducens) nucleus** and its connections.

I plainly see the nucleus; the internal facial genu wraps around it. But I know that it's intimately associated with **paramedian pontine reticular formation**, about which several observations come to mind:

1. It's not readily visualized (it's reticular);
2. It's present both at the level of CN VI nucleus and above/rostral to CN VI nucleus;
3. If you can't readily visualize it, how do you know where it is? In young monkeys, stimulation by an electrode passed from rostral to caudal in brainstem resulted in (Cohen et al., 1968):

    a. vocalization at the level of central grey matter surrounding aqueduct of Sylvius;
    b. depression of one eye in adduction (intorsion of the eye contralateral to the site of stimulation) at the level of CN IV nucleus;

c. adduction of one eye (the eye ipsilateral to the site of stimulation) at the level of medial longitudinal fasciculus above CN VI nucleus);
   d. conjugate, ipsilateral, horizontal eye movements when in the paramedian pontine reticular formation (if stimulation on the left, then both eyes look horizontally to the left);
4. It's involved in gaze holding;
5. If you *lesion* it (say, in the left paramedian pontine reticular formation), you cause paresis or paralysis of conjugate, ipsilateral, horizontal gaze (both eyes can't look horizontally to the left).

So, how do you differentiate between a lesion of (left) paramedian pontine reticular formation, a lesion of (left) CN VI nucleus itself, a lesion of fascicles emerging from (left) CN VI but still within the pons, and a (left) CN VI palsy?

The four parts of the question yield four distinct answers, each of which requires anatomical information.

Regarding (left) **paramedian pontine reticular formation**, I read that it's "the final prenuclear anatomical substrate for ipsilateral saccades" (Daroff et al., 1990). What do those words mean *in detail*? With respect to a cortically directed horizontal saccade of both eyes *to the left*, one typically invokes the so-called frontal eye field *in right cortex*–roughly, the posterior portion of the right middle frontal gyrus. One could also talk about a role for *right* superior colliculus as well, since right frontal eye field also projects to right superior colliculus by way of so-called "direct" and "indirect" basal ganglionic pathways.

Decussation of the corticobulbar pathway to left brainstem is said to happen somewhere in the reticular formation, either at the level of low midbrain or upper pons. At the level of the decussation, we are supra- or pre-nuclear, relative to CN VI nucleus. The corticobulbar projection, specifically with respect to our horizontal saccade of both eyes to the left, terminates in left paramedian pontine reticular formation, which is the location of excitatory burst neurons that project to two types of CN VI neurons. A lesion in paramedian pontine reticular formation–and one has as yet really to describe [left] CN VI nucleus–results in a paralysis of conjugate lateral gaze to the left.

(Left) **CN VI nucleus** isn't same as the paramedian pontine reticular formation. Fascicles leaving the nucleus emerge from its medial aspect en route to their exit as the abducens nerve at ventral pons. (In an appropriately stained axial section, it's easy to confuse CN VI fascicles as part of the internal facial genu, but those two differ, of course.) The nucleus contains not only motoneurons related to its control of the lateral rectus muscle, but also internuclear neurons whose fibers cross the midline roughly at the level of (left) CN VI nucleus to ascend in right medial longitudinal fasciculus. To repeat, interneurons inside (left) CN VI nucleus receive excitatory bursts from the (left) paramedian pontine reticular formation just as the motoneurons do.

The nucleus *receives* afferents not only from (left) pontine paramedian reticular formation, but also: from the (left) inner ear vestibule via (left) medial vestibular nucleus, (left) vestibular sensory ganglion of Scarpa (which is uniquely situated within CN VIII), and from the nucleus prepositus hypoglossi, which we'll discuss when we get to medulla in chapter 12.

Daroff et al. (1990) write that ". . . a unilateral lesion of the sixth nucleus produces an ipsilateral gaze palsy"; *both* eyes can't move to the left, because we know about interneurons inside CN VI nucleus. The authors make a further point, specifically with respect to a CN VI nuclear lesion, that "the *almost obligate* ipsilateral facial palsy, caused by involvement of the facial nerve fascicle dorsal to the nucleus, *provides the only reliable clinical means of distinguishing this gaze palsy from that produced by a PPRF [paramedian pontine reticular formation] lesion at the same level* [my italics]."

Next, regarding **fascicles emerging from (left) CN VI but still within the pons**, Carpenter and Sutin (1983) write: "[t]he abducens [nucleus] appears to be the only motor cranial nerve in which disturbances with lesions of root fibers and nucleus are not identical." Here's why: a nuclear lesion looks like a lesion of the paramedian pontine reticular formation, not like a mononeuropathy affecting (left) lateral rectus in isolation. And, as we just read, a nuclear lesion characteristically involves the fascicles of the facial genu, hence the complete facial palsy described in the case that began this chapter. From the original 1858 report, we read:

> . . . while he tries to move both or each separately, the eyes at once appear in the middle of the interpalpebral space to stop without being able to pass over [to the left] (Foville, 1858, translation by Silverman et al., 1995).[2]

And, yes, his left face was paralyzed as if he had a Bell's palsy.

The CN VI fascicle or "central rootlet" leaving the medial side of the nucleus passes through the entire pontine tegmentum and basis pontis before it exits the brainstem. A fascicular CN VI lesion, like a fascicular CN VII lesion, shares many clinical aspects of an extra-axial cranial nerve palsy. But given that the fascicle *en passant* keeps company with many other structures, a (left) pontine lesion can produce signs in addition to a (left) lateral rectus palsy, like a contralateral (right body) hemiparesis among many other possible findings.

Regarding **an isolated (left) CN VI palsy**, we'd expect an isolated paresis of (left eye) abduction in the horizontal plane without an associated adduction problem in the right eye.

*

You're interested to address how the third of three findings from the 1858 case, the hemiparesis in the *right* body, links up with the first two findings.

I beg for patience until chapter 11, just a few pages away.

*

We're still standing atop the facial colliculi. Indeed you're wondering if we ever plan to move elsewhere. Yet from this vantage point, thinking

---

[2] For the record, the Foville in question, author of the 1858 case, was Achille Louis François Foville (1832-1887), not his father, who was Achille Louis Foville (1799-1878). Both were anatomists and clinicians (Brogna et al., 2012).

truly three dimensionally (**RULE #3**), we can appreciate the great deal that's all around us.

I am interested in what might be lateral to the facial colliculus, moving across the floor of the fourth ventricle. The dome of the facial colliculus ends. At its lateral base angle, there's another mound extending to the lateral edge of the fourth ventricle. That mound, described as a vestibular triangle (Nauta and Feirtag, 1986), contains, yes, vestibular nuclei.

There's a tendency for some to think of vestibular nuclei as being located just in the medulla. They're there in fact, but a column created by vestibular nuclei (no less than four nuclei) extends rostrally to our current level of pons. Since a fundamental task of the vestibular system is to control eye movements relative to the head's position in space, it makes sense that vestibular nuclei would be anatomically close to sites we've already discussed relevant to saccades and gaze.

I like to think much more simply: the vestibular nuclear column that extends, without interruption, from medulla to pons is . . . sensory. Anatomists say that the vestibular axons from vestibular nuclei are the most widely dispersed special sensory system in the neuraxis. They dispatch themselves to brainstem motor nuclei (especially those having to do with eyes), to cerebellum (especially vestibulocerebellum[3] or the flocculus and nodulus), to spinal cord, and to thalamus thence to cortex (Carpenter and Sutin, 1983 and Nieuwenhuys et al., 2008), but the nuclei themselves live in a single, discrete column.

Deep and lateral to the vestibular-nuclear column in the vestibular triangle, might we expect to find another sensory nucleus? Yes: **the spinal tract and nucleus of CN V**–it's a structure that we can track caudally into medulla and to cervical spinal cord (basically, it's a column).

Medial to spinal tract and nucleus of CN V, and medial to the vestibular nuclear column, would we expect other sensory nuclei? No, not if you're a proponent of a limiting sulcus that divides motor from

---

[3] Rather than "vestibulocerebellum," some anatomists prefer the term "oculomotor cerebellum," which consists of more than just flocculus and nodulus.

sensory nuclei in pons. Instead, you'd expect motor nuclei, among them CN VI and CN VII motor nuclei (CN V motor nucleus is also medial, but it's located in the higher pons, as discussed in the last chapter) and **superior salivatory nucleus**, which is secreto*motor*. You find them where they, um, belong.

*

If I reach up to touch the fourth ventricle's fastigium (top) above me, previously my fingers touched the under side of the superior medullary velum and the lingula above it, but, now, buried in an expanse of white matter are **deep cerebellar nuclei**, the largest and most lateral of which is the **dentate nucleus**. Depending on the transverse section, perhaps a bit of vestibulocerebellar **nodulus** pokes into the dorsal space of fourth ventricle above my head.

To either side of my outstretched arms, the margins of the ventricle still angle inwards, relative to the undulated fourth ventricular floor. Yet, it's not just the superior cerebellar peduncle/brachium conjunctivum and middle cerebellar peduncle/brachium pontis that envelop me here. Once I visualize in my head the vestibular nuclear cell column in the vestibular triangle, since I know that some vestibular efferents from all four vestibular nuclei pass to cerebellum, I know I'm in the vicinity of the **juxtarestiform body**, through which those vestibulocerebellar fibers pass.

The juxtarestiform body lies at the dorsomedial edge of the **restiform body** or **inferior cerebellar peduncle**. (In a lateral view of an intact brainstem at the level of the medulla, the inferior cerebellar peduncle resembles a rope or, in Latin, a *restis* that passes from spinal cord upwards towards cerebellum, hence the alternative name.)

It's only in the pons where you visualize all three cerebellar peduncles in one transverse section. All three peduncles can be found in the white matter that I touch with my laterally outstretched arms.

*

Ventral to the floor of fourth ventricle, we re-acknowledge white matter tracts we've already encountered:

> **medial longitudinal fasciculus** at the midline, below my feet;
> **tectospinal tract**, just below the medial longitudinal fasciculus, retaining its intimate proximity to it;
> **central tegmental tract**;
> **spinothalamic and medial lemniscal tracts**, ventral to the central tegmental tract;
> and, dorsolaterally, **lateral lemniscus**;
> the **pyramidal tracts** in the ventral basis pontis.

There's something almost too obvious about the pons:

> The pons itself is riddled with fascicles. The transverse ones are pontocerebellar fibers, which cross the midline to join the contralateral brachium pontis. The longitudinal ones are corticopontine, corticobulbar, and corticospinal. The tegmentum—the dorsal division of the section—includes motor nuclei, sensory cell groups, and the reticular core of the section. It also includes nearly all of the brainstem's long fiber systems (Nauta and Feirtag, 1986).

I think that a conscientious student has some sense about which tracts run up and down as opposed to side to side, but there are opportunities to become confused. In an axial section in which white matter stains darkly, two transversely oriented black smears on either side of the midline separate the dorsal pontine tegmentum from the ventral basis pontis. In real anatomical dimensions, the thick white matter of those smears can be found just 0.75 centimeters below the floor of the fourth ventricle. Their transverse orientation shouldn't confuse, because we know that the **medial lemniscus** changes its axis during its winding brainstem course (in the pons it is transverse), but it's a longitudinal fiber system and an obvious pontine structure. But the black smears aren't exclusively the medial lemnisci.

Less anatomically obvious is the **anterolateral fasciculus** (the **spinothalamic tract**), which is just lateral to the medial lemniscus; it, too, is a longitudinal fiber system. The **lateral lemniscus**, also a longitudinal fiber system and also found (dorso)lateral to medial lemniscus, heads to **inferior colliculus** in the auditory pathway. Yet the **trapezoid body** runs from side to side: its fibers cross the midline transversely and bidirectionally just at the place (or, ever so slightly inferior to) where we visualize the medial lemnisci as sideways smears. The trapezoid body is also part of the auditory pathway, and its anatomical presence introduces a curiosity in any attempt to organize one's thinking about the brainstem along the lines of a basal and alar plate division.

*

A few paragraphs ago, I asked, "Medial to spinal tract and nucleus of CN V, and medial to the vestibular nuclear column, would we expect other sensory nuclei?" I said that we wouldn't. But now consider a nucleus that is related and very proximate to the trapezoid body.

Buried in the stained, white-matter blackness of trapezoid body is a **superior olive**. I've traced the auditory pathway more completely in a monograph on language (Miyawaki, 2018b), but for our present purposes, let me note: a. the superior olive is a key nucleus that receives auditory information from both cochleas; b. in an atlas of human brainstem, the superior olive can be hard to point to; c. I had never understood how it looked like an "olive" (such as the inferior olive) until I looked into the auditory pathways of mammals like bats, cats, or dogs. In the cat, for example, there's no mistaking a resemblance between superior olive and inferior olive. A convoluted, twisting shape of superior olivary nucleus is found in some mammals, but not in humans (Moore, 1987 and Nieuwenhuys et al., 2008).

The superior olive–actually, it's a complex of nuclei–is *medial* to the facial motor nucleus in the pontine tegmentum. Isn't it a sensory nucleus as CN VIII is a sensory nerve? Nieuwenhuys (2011) describes superior olive as a "center of higher order." Is he blurring a basal-alar division that he takes so seriously?

*

Warning, I end this long chapter with an aside based on a dated reference (Irving and Harrison, 1967).

What possesses someone to perform a study in 49 mammals representing 14 species in which, among other goals, one wants to compare, for each species, the number of cells in a subnucleus of superior olive against the number of cells in CN VI nucleus? It turns out that there's a linear relationship, very convincing in animals with predominantly rod retinas, between the number of cells in medial superior olivary subnucleus and in CN VI nucleus. The authors factored nuclear diameters in relation to thickness of sections to arrive at estimated neuronal numbers. In the cat (large medial superior olive; rod retina), for example, there are about 1,000 neurons in CN VI nucleus and over 4,000 in medial superior olive. In the rat (small medial superior olive; rod retina), by comparison, there are roughly 200 neurons in CN VI nucleus compared to 700 in medial superior olive.

In animals with cone foveas or retinas, there's a similar linear relationship: the greater the number of superior olivary neurons, the greater the number of neurons in CN VI nucleus. In the macaque (large medial superior olive, cone fovea), the numbers are: roughly 4,500 CN VI neurons and just under 3,500 medial superior olivary neurons.

In ten species with rod retinas, there's no linear relationship between cell counts in CN VI nucleus and different auditory nucleus located in trapezoid body.

The linear relationship specifically with respect to superior olive, the authors wrote, support a notion that there's an aspect of the auditory system ". . . probably concerned with the control of the visual apparatus by the location (and probably other aspects) of sounds. This system is present in animals with large eyes and may be regarded as a visual auditory system, having evolved as an adjunct of vision."

Is the quote a description of "higher-order" processing? One starts to wonder what a sensory nucleus really is—or in what way there might be nuclei most properly designated "sensorimotor."

11.

What About the Weakness?
"L'hémiplégie alterne"[4]

At last, what's to be made of the 43-year-old man's right hemiparesis together with his conjugate left gaze palsy and left facial palsy? I want us to think . . . long before we blurt the words "left pons."

Recall from last chapter that the man's event happened early in the morning on June 17, 1858. By June 29, twelve or so days later, the gaze palsy and facial weakness were unchanged, but his right hemiparesis improved such that he could walk without help. The patient had an atrophy of the right arm antedating his event, so Foville was tentative to conclude much about the arm. I can't find a comment or hint about a sensory disturbance at any point. My French is rudimentary.

But it's still good enough to read that crossed hemipareses (right body, left face or vice versa) had been discussed at the Paris Anatomical Society for some years before 1858. The pons had the been contemplated

---

[4] Weakness doesn't alternate from one side of the body to the other, as it does in, say, in the alternating hemiplegia of childhood, a pediatric genetic syndrome. It's a bit unfortunate that some authors talk about Foville and other eponymic brainstem syndromes as "alternating hemipareses" (e.g., Carpenter and Sutin, 1983). As Foville specifies, *"alterne"* really means *"une paralysie d'un côté du corps et du côté opposé de la face* [a paralysis of one side of the body and the opposite side of the face]."

as the site of causative lesions in *l'hémiplégie alterne* by many, including Poisson, Sénac, Millard, Gubler, Grenet, and perhaps even in his own father's textbook, from which Foville quotes.

Fast forward to this century and my hospital. Colleagues published a teaching case in 2006 (Selvadurai et al, 2006), in which we read that "a 68-year-old man with a pontine telangiectasia on anticoagulation developed a left conjugate gaze palsy and right hemiparesis." In an accompanying video, the right arm is obviously weak and a left conjugate gaze palsy is also clear. There's no comment about the leg. There's no left facial paresis. Imaging showed an acute pontine hemorrhage extending dorsally and to the left. The left facial colliculus seems in the territory of the bleed. In a hemorrhage, you could argue that blood, unlike an ischemic infarction, might spare some structures, perhaps the left internal facial genu in particular.

Question: there's no pathological correlation to Foville's case, so how does one definitively explain *either* an incomplete presentation (as in 2006) *or* the complete one of 1858?

*

Let's speculate that the 43 year old suffered just a right monoparesis of the leg (which improved), just as the 68 year old seems to exhibit just a right arm monoparesis. Or, let's say that the 43 year old acutely suffered both arm and leg weakness, even if Foville couldn't tell with certainty because of the congenital deficit. Can we address the anatomy in all three permutations?

Given that somatotopic organization can be found in many nuclei and tracts throughout the neuraxis, the results of a prospective study correlating clinical and imaging findings might surprise:

> Despite the high number of pontine infarctions, we could not find any significant difference in pontine lesion location between patients with a predominantly arm paresis and those with a predominantly leg paresis. There was an area significantly affected by lesions

causing arm predominant hemiparesis in the pons, but the lesions causing leg paresis appeared to be located above, within, and below it . . . (Marx et al., 2005).

The authors were interested in patients with acute oculomotor disorders, cranial nerve dysfunction, and limb or gait abnormalities suggestive of acute posterior circulation dysfunction. They recruited 258 consecutive patients; all were MR imaged within 48 hours of their events. Forty-one were diagnosed with something aside from a brainstem infarction.

Of the remaining 217, 155 had MR-diagnosed brainstem infarcts. Among the 155, 44 suffered an acute motor hemiparesis; 111 did not. Three of the 44 had multiple brainstem infarcts and were excluded. The remaining 41, all with isolated lesions and motor hemipareses, were used for correlation analysis. Clinically ascertained deficits were also studied with motor-evoked-potential studies within a week of presentation, save in three instances.

Of 41 motor hemipareses, arm weakness (more than leg) occurred in 20, leg weakness (more than arm) in 7; in 14 cases, arm and leg weakness were comparable. Three-dimensional image reconstructions and statistical analysis found: in a comparison of the 111 patients without hemiparesis and the 41 with hemiparesis, ventromedial, upper pontine lesions correlated with contralateral weakness of all types. Arm weakness mapped to pons at a level a bit superior to the level of the facial colliculus. Leg weakness mapped to levels above, at, and below the arm region.

We don't know much about the components of *l'hémiplégie alterne* in individual cases. All we know is that 14 of 41 had a facial paresis; 8 of 41 had some form of unspecified oculomotor disorder. We don't know how many had facial paresis and a conjugate gaze palsy together.

In their discussion, the authors sound ever so slightly apologetic: ". . . at least a moderate degree of corticospinal tract somatotopy is still maintained in the pons" even if (quoting from earlier in the text) "based on primate lesion studies . . . topographic arm/leg distribution appears to be progressively lost as the descending [corticospinal] tract traverses the pons."

They arrived at conclusions they didn't expect.

Save for arm paresis (maybe), pontine localization at a specific level based on weakness alone isn't as precise as the localization of a (left) conjugate lateral gaze palsy. And even a lesion at (left) facial colliculus can still produce an incomplete syndrome, as the 2006 teaching case attests.

*

The correlation paper is refreshing, because it reminds us that clinical data are . . . just what they are. When studying textbook anatomy, it's easy to be interrupted by Monday-morning questions, among them (my curt responses are in brackets):

> Why wouldn't there be facial sensory manifestations and contralateral hemibody sensory manifestations in Foville's *l'hémiplégie alterne*? [Maybe there were.]
>
> Could the hemiparesis in the 43 year old have been an ataxic hemiparesis (which improved)? [Yes.]
>
> Why wasn't there even a suggestion of left facial paresis in the teaching case from 2006? [We've kinda answered that one.]
>
> Assuming the 1858 case was an ischemic stroke, how large was the ischemic territory? [We'll never know.]
>
> If it's true that somatotopy fractures (becomes somehow disorganized) in the pons, why is that? [Dunno. For that matter, why is there fractured somatotopy all through the cerebellum?]

Even if hemiparesis had not been present in the 43 year old's case, there's reason to believe that A.L.F. Foville, all of 26 years old and a year out of medical school, would still have written his paper. The first words of his publication's title reveal his almost naive, absolutely central interest: *"Note sur une paralysie peu connue de certains muscles de l'œil* . . . [Note on a little-known paralysis of some muscles of the eye]." He had no knowledge of the paramedian pontine reticular formation and its burst neurons, of the two types of neurons in CN VI nucleus, and, most importantly, he had no familiarity with the medial longitudinal fasciculus, because its existence was unknown at the time. He was fascinated by the conjugate gaze palsy.

Pons associated with *l'hémiplégie alterne* was old hat to him.

*

We can amplify *alterne* to apply to brainstem as a whole, not just to pons.

A _____ of one side of the body and a _____ on the opposite side of the face makes one think about a brainstem localization, for which, as always, there are three possible answers.

"Face" means almost anything about it: the (left) eye, (left) pupil, (left) eyelid, the (left and right) eyes (looking to the left), (left) facial strength or sensation, (left) palate, (left) tongue, or what have you. And the contralateral hemibody findings are no less possibly diverse: (right) paresis, (right) ataxia, (right) paresthesiae, (right) sensory loss, (right) tremor, or what have you.

You want to see some *alterne* aspect to localize a lesion in brainstem. But the findings especially in the face–see the last paragraph for a definition of "face"–allow you, as a matter of principle, to increase your 0.333 likelihood of diagnostic success to a number approximating one.

12.

Folded Grey Mass

The moment I visualize even a part of the folded grey mass that is **inferior olive**, I know that I'm in medulla. This chapter's title is from Brodal (1981). He reminds us that we refer to an obvious *collection of neurons* in the neighborhood of (depending on the cut, dorsal or lateral to) the medullary pyramid.

Not all axial sections in atlases are perfectly transverse. At the pontomedullary junction, which is our location now, sometimes you see just a sliver of inferior olive on one side but not the other. Not to worry.

*

RULE #7: If inferior olive anywhere, then medulla there.

*

I've seen students confuse inferior olive with another folded grey mass found in the vast, deep cerebellar white matter dorsal to the fourth ventricle. The latter grey matter is dentate nucleus, which we've encountered previously. There's reason to associate dentate nucleus and inferior olive in one's mind, because one could consider inferior olive as a ventrally displaced cerebellar nucleus (Kahle, 1986).

Pause. Think back to chapter 8, where we discussed output from cerebellum:

> The superior cerebellar peduncle is the largest efferent tract leaving cerebellum; it's an arm that bends in space to reach across the midline. Its axons (say, in the right brachium conjunctivum) arise from (right) dentate nucleus, the most lateral of the (right) deep cerebellar nuclei. The (right) superior cerebellar peduncle connects (right) deep cerebellar nuclei with red nucleus and, mainly, with thalamus on the contralateral (left) side.

The dentate is an important output nucleus (output from cerebellum via superior cerebellar peduncle a.k.a. brachium conjunctivum, to contralateral brain). The inferior olive is also an output nucleus–this chapter helps to fill the following blank–to contralateral _____?

*

The inferior olive is conspicuous. In humans, it's . . . beautiful.

Let's elaborate. The **principal nucleus of inferior olive** is especially well developed in humans, much more so than in a rat or cat (Baizer et al., 2011). There are two other subdivisions of inferior olive, including a dorsal accessory olive and a medial accessory olive, but I'll discuss the principal nucleus in particular. Its infoldings and sheer size distinguish it from other grey structures of brainstem. Thinking in three dimensions, an old anatomist described it as a "crumpled purse" whose opening is the **hilus**.

White matter cloaks the principal nucleus: the **central tegmental tract** "forms a fleece of myelinated fibres around the olive" (Nieuwenhuys et al., 2008); the fleece is the inferior olive's **amiculum** (cloak).

*

Perhaps you've noticed that textbook diagrams of cerebellar Purkinje cells depict just one climbing fiber per Purkinje cell. The origin of "the one" climbing fiber per Purkinje cell is inferior olive. Here's a good description:

> The fibers arising from the inferior olive end by branching on to the main neurons of the cerebellar cortex[,] called the Purkinje cells. These are the largest nerve cells in the brain, and the ends of the inferior olive axons, termed climbing fibers, literally climb up over the Purkinje cells' branching dendrites (fingerlike projections providing additional surface), where neurons receive input from other neurons (Llinás, 2001).

Other input to the Purkinje dendritic tree—by way of mossy fibers, not climbing fibers—includes, for example, cerebral cortical input via pontine nuclei and middle cerebellar peduncle. (Recall again from chapter 8: the middle cerebellar peduncle is the largest afferent pathway into cerebellum, "quantitatively the most important route by which the cerebral cortex can influence cerebellar cortex.") Purkinje axons, in turn, project to deep cerebellar nuclei, the dentate being the largest among them.

What's to be made of an architectural similarity between cerebral cortex, cerebellar cortex, the (highly folded) principal nucleus of inferior olive, and (also highly folded) dentate nucleus? Baizer et al. (2011) wonder about an evolutionary significance to involution or convolution of grey matter: ". . . human IOpr [principal nucleus of inferior olive] is reminiscent of the expansion of both cerebral and cerebellar cortex, both of which remain sheets with the development of sulci and gyri and a complex folding pattern. The increase in folding in the IOpr is similar to what is seen in the human dentate nucleus. Cerebral and cerebellar cortex, the IOpr, and the dentate nucleus all show complex folding patterns [in humans] . . .."

Not all grey matter structures involute, as Rakic (1995) pondered: cortical surface area increases by orders of magnitude from mouse to human, but cortical thickness only doubles between the species; then, if one compares the macaque monkey and human, asks Rakic,

"What is the explanation for the approximately 15-fold larger number of postmitotic cells becoming distributed in the form of a thin, regular [folded] sheet rather than in a lump or globe, as has occurred during enlargement of the neostriatum over the same evolutionary period?"

The skeptic asks: so what?

The anatomist says: foldedness isn't just beautiful; it's very human.

In a pathway we'll trace in a moment, principal nucleus of inferior olive projects to cerebellar hemisphere, specifically to Purkinje cells. Brodal (1981) begs to differ about a one-to-one relationship between olivary and cerebellar cells: "It is often stated that there is a specific relation of one climbing fiber to one Purkinje cell. . .. [A]natomically, branching of climbing fibers has been seen only in or just beneath the [cerebellar] cortex, and these branches supply two, three, or four Purkinje cells not far removed from each other. . . physiological investigations show that a single climbing fiber may branch and supply folia that are considerable distances apart." It appears that I've mis-taught all these years about one climbing fiber per Purkinje cell–maybe an excusable error.

What route do inferior olivary axons take to become climbing fibers specific to Purkinje cells?

*

The reader has noticed that I idiosyncratically situate myself in places like fourth ventricle. In the medulla, I'll start inside the **anterior median fissure**, my head above/dorsal to my feet. It's a tight space. I'm curious to know what's above me, close to the midline on either side, all the way up to the floor of the fourth ventricle.

We've not encountered the anterior median fissure. Neither have we really seen the medullary pyramids themselves, because the advent of a pyramid as a visible enlargement of ventroanterior funiculus *means* the medulla, along with the appearance of inferior olive lateral to pyramid. Because the ventroanterior funiculi on the ventral surface of medulla so robustly enlarge, the anterior median fissure between pyramids results, and that fissure extends all the way caudal/down to the point where it's briefly effaced by the decussation of the pyramids at the cervicomedullary junction.

Inside the anterior median fissure, to the immediate right and left of me, are the pyramids, but not just the pyramids.

Warning, here's a digression, but worth the trouble. In an appropriately stained section, the pyramids are black (all white matter), but there's space around the pyramids that isn't black. In fact, there are also *nuclei* to the immediate left and right of me in the anterior median fissure. In the spirit of "what *is* that?" (last asked in chapter 6), I looked into those **arcuate nuclei**, which really do "curve" from the medial aspect of the pyramid, then ventral to it, then lateral to it.

Come to discover that the arcuate nuclei are part of a medullary serotonergic network involved in control of the internal milieu, particularly its respiratory aspects (Kinney et al., 2011). For all the time in my life spent listening to patterns of breath in stuporous or comatose patients, I had no idea whatsoever about a role for nuclei I barely noticed in my books. You can see for yourself in a good atlas: they're obviously there.[5]

---

[5] To illustrate how widespread arcuate nuclear connections might be, try a dissection:

Look at the dorsal side of a medulla, particularly at the lower/caudal half of the fourth ventricle tented by the **inferior medullary velum**. Remove that velum to examine the floor of the fourth ventricle. You'll see a variable number of transversely running fibers which mark a kind of horizontal midline between the upper fourth ventricle and the end of the fourth ventricle, the latter called the **obex**.

The beautiful lateral strands, first observed by Piccolomini in the 16th century (Swanson, 2015), have been thought to be acoustic or cerebellar in nature, but a tracer study (Zec et al., 1997) suggests that arcuate nuclei project up the midline raphe and on to the floor of the fourth ventricle as these **medullary striae of Piccolomini**. The striae end in the vicinity of the inferior cerebellar peduncles at the level of the **foraminae of Luschka**. Also from the arcuate nuclei, passing superficially and laterally over the pyramids and olives, so-called **external arcuate fibers** end at much the same lateral place. Exposure to cerebrospinal fluid (for both projections) might relate to the homeostatic function of the network.

A midline seam dividing left and right halves of medulla points directly at the top of my head. On either side of the seam are white matter tracts that are, at a glance, parallel to the seam. Their fibers run from below to above where I stand. The **medial lemniscus**, as we know, changes axis along its ribbon-like course heading rostrally. Here the medial lemnisci are "upright," if you glean my meaning. I've characterized the medial lemnisci in my classes as a headless person *standing upon* the pyramids–headless, because there's no representation of the head at our current level; arm representation in either lemniscus is above leg (arm higher than leg in each hemibody representation). Such are the up-standing medial lemnisci, but if I think carefully, the white matter above me can't just be passing in the caudal to rostral direction. There's a cross-weave of fibers above me.

Dorsolateral to the pyramid on either side is the principal nucleus of inferior olive, whose hilus points towards the midline. Inferior olivary axons emerge from the hilum, and pass transversely–for illustration, from (right) hilus, *across* (right) medial lemniscus, then across the midline seam, then *across* (left) medial lemniscus. The fibers travel at right angles to the up-down fibers of the lemnisci, heading to contralateral destinations. Where?

Verbose answers:

1. The fibers traverse to (left) **inferior cerebellar peduncle**, a.k.a. the (left) **restiform body**, which is present very laterally at our axial level. The inferior cerebellar peduncles look like large, thick commas on either side, per Nauta (1986), but they're buried in other (middle cerebellar) peduncular or deep cerebellar white matter.
    1a. By the way, **olivocerebellar fibers** constitute the largest component of inferior cerebellar peduncle (Carpenter and Sutin, 1983).
2. **Via** (left) **inferior cerebellar peduncle**, axons pass, now as climbing fibers, to (left) **cerebellar hemisphere** in the case of

(right) principal nucleus of the inferior olive, specifically to the **Purkinje cell layer**.

3. If we consider other inferior olivary subnuclei, their axons arrive at other cerebellar/Purkinje-cell-layer destinations (e.g., **medial accessory olive** to **flocculus** and **vermis**; you might be interested to know that the medial accessory olive is especially developed in the sonar-savvy porpoise, compared to humans [Baizer et al., 2011]).

*

What's dorsal to **medial lemniscus** above my head? Moving ventral to dorsal, we've identified these structures previously:

> **central tegmental tract**, a bit lateral to the medial lemnisci; it ends in medulla as the **amiculum of the inferior olive**;
> **tectospinal tract**, which retains its intimate proximity to medial longitudinal fasciculus, then:
> **medial longitudinal fasciculus**.

We're quite not done. At our axial level, dorsal to the medial longitudinal fasciculus, are nuclei just under the floor of the fourth ventricle on either side of the midline seam. Their location tempts one to think of some motor function akin to other, very midline nuclei (think CN IV nuclei for example), but what *are* they?

*

> **RULE #8**: If you're in medulla, and if you see midline nuclei just ventral to the floor of the fourth ventricle, then DON'T assume that you've found the hypoglossal nuclei.

*

Maybe we could call them nuclei *presiding* over the hypoglossal nuclei, since we're now above/higher than the level of the hypoglossal (CN XII) nuclei. So be it, since the same thought occurred to anatomists a long time ago, but let's use Latin.

The vertical distance between CN VI nuclei and CN XII nuclei is filled by the column-shaped **nucleus prepositus hypoglossi** on either side of the midline (McCrea and Horn, 2006). It's a nucleus of interneurons; it's involved in the control of eye movements probably *not* by way of projections into near-by medial longitudinal fasciculus (McCrea and Baker, 1985).[6] Its interneurons connect to and/or from many nodes, among them: vestibular nuclei, paramedian pontine reticular formation, inferior olive, flocculus, nodulus, vermis, superior colliculus, thalamus, and extraocular motor nuclei. I have abbreviated the list; there are other start and end points related to this curiously central structure.

---

[6] We should probably disabuse ourselves of the notion that the medial longitudinal fasciculus is the only avenue that connects vestibular nuclei to ocular motor nuclei. The connections of the nucleus prepositus hypoglossi are an example, as is the **ascending tract of Deiters**, which is an excitatory pathway from medial vestibular nucleus to CN III nucleus. Without crossing the midline, it ascends lateral to the medial longitudinal fasciculus.

13.

Oblivious to Ocular Lateropulsion

Some years ago, residents in our program asked whether I could review a few years of Residency In-Training Examinations, distill all prior questions related to neuroanatomy, then give a talk about what trainees needed to know for the next exam. At least they were honest about what they wanted.

In prepping for the lecture, I ran across the term "ocular lateropulsion."

Taking a break from axial sections, I'll ask now: what is it?

1. Let's start with normality. Open both eyes, look straight ahead, perhaps at some distant object directly in front of you. Now close your eyes for a few seconds. Now, open them. Are your eyes still fixed on the object? If yes, then we'll call that normal.
2. Now consider the phenomenon. The patient seems relaxed, as relaxed as one can be while being examined. You instruct her to look straight ahead.

What if her eyes don't look, to you, exactly straight ahead? You're not sure, but it seems as if she's gazing at something off to one side. The deviation could be subtle; it could be obvious.

I'm not discussing anything like a skew deviation or anything else but a sense that the eyes don't quite look straight ahead.[7]

3. You ask her, "are you looking straight ahead?" She says, "yup."
4. We'll have her close her eyes for a few seconds. In that interval, her eyes conjugately roam to one side in the horizontal plane. We know, because when she opens her eyes, they are deviated incompletely or very completely to one side. Regardless, they have moved without question, "lateropulsed."

In a series of 14 consecutive cases reported in 1974 (all with ocular lateropulsion), we read:

> The lateral deviation in all cases appeared when the patients were requested to relax and "gaze straight ahead." *All* patients were quite unaware of the lateral deviation (with the exception of one . . . [whose eyes "were locked" to the right side]); to reach the midposition of the eyes they had voluntarily to deviate the eyes in the opposite direction. Some patients, however, were not able to maintain *a* position of steady, voluntary straight-forward or contralateral gaze. In six patients . . . the tonic pull could be overcome only for *a* very short while. When they were requested to keep the gaze in a direction opposite to the conjugate deviation, the eyes slowly drifted away to the tonically deviated position. The drift was characteristically smooth "*as if the eyeballs were pulled by elastic bands*"; it was

---

[7] Lateropulsion and skew deviation aren't mutually exclusive. Regarding the latter, the following is useful: "In typical skew deviations, the higher eye is contralateral to a medullary lesion and ipsilateral to a mid pontine (the level at which otolith projections decussate the brainstem) or midbrain lesion. . . . in the case of a left lateral medullary syndrome, an ocular tilt reaction might involve left head tilt, right hyperdeviation, and counterroll of the eyes (upper poles) toward the left shoulder . . ." (Frohman et al., 2008). But in my vignette, I'm interested in a clue that lateropulsion will occur when fixation is lost–i.e., when she closes her eyes.

occasionally interrupted by rapid and large nystagmoid beats in the direction of attempted voluntary gaze . . . [emphases are original to the paper] (Hörnsten, 1974b).

The above is worth parsing. Why? Because there's relevance especially to the medulla. Also because, if we don't read the passage with care, we'll miss something stunning.

The 14 cases weren't instances of a conjugate gaze palsy like that described our chapter 10. They *were* able to get the eyes past the midline . . . in the direction opposite to the lateropulsion. It might have been effortful, but still possible: some weren't able to maintain *a* position of steady, voluntary straight-forward or contralateral gaze; or, the elastic-band pull could be overcome only briefly; but conjugate gaze to the side opposite the lateropulsion was doable.

Why were *all* patients, save the one whose eyes *locked* to one side, "quite unaware of the lateral deviation"? They were unaware or oblivious, because, from their point of view, they looked straight ahead.

Is there a sense in which the idea of *what's straight ahead* changes?

By the way, the 14 cases were all medullary infarctions. As a rule of thumb, the direction of lateropulsion pointed to the side of the lesion.

*

Let's experiment on our normal selves again.

1. There's a tree with a big trunk in a nearby park. It stands alone without anything around it. The trunk is tilted a bit against the snowy ground of winter.
2. We wonder if it's possible to make the trunk look straight up and down. It tilts to the right, maybe by 10 degrees.
3. We tilt our head about 10 degrees to our right; does that make the trunk straight? I tried it. My answer is: I can sorta make it look straight, but I know it's not. How do I know?

4. We recall from physics that, assuming a mass isn't influenced by other masses, it falls in a plumb vertical line in a gravitational field.
5. How do I know the vertical line in the gravitational field in the park? It's actually that vertical line which allows me to conclude that the tree trunk tilts in space. The tilt is relative to the verticality. Tilting my head doesn't help.
6. There's an objective vertical which generally matches what has been called the subjective visual vertical.

Quoting again from the series of 14 cases, "*Torsion of the visual fields* [author's emphasis] was initially experienced by three patients.... This phenomenon was very dramatic in [two] patients, who felt as if the surroundings were tilted 180° for the first few minutes. A 90° tilt persisted in [one] patient for several days" (Hörnsten, 1974a). A subjective visual vertical at odds with the objective vertical as determined by gravity occurs in brainstem pathology, particular medullary pathology (Dieterich and Brandt, 1993).

Some argue that paroxysmal "tilts" of the world differ from actual measurements of the subjective visual vertical:

> ... a pathologic "tilt illusion," in which the world is seen to be on its side or inverted, is experienced transiently by patients with lateral medullary, thalamic, or even cerebral infarct or hemorrhage. However, central or peripheral lesions typically do not cause complaints of an abnormal sense of the vertical, and any disturbance goes undetected unless patients are tested when deprived of visual information [they are tested in darkness] (Sharpe, 2003, an editorial regarding Bronstein et al., 2003).

"Goes undetected" is my interest in the passage. You can't *not* detect a sensation of environment tilt: up becomes down and vice versa. In reported series, there are variations–90° tilts, etc. (Sierra-Hidalgo et al., 2012). Yet, ever so subtly and without personal awareness, a sense of "straight ahead" and of gravity's true axis can change in a medullary disease process.

Subjective perception sounds redundant (what perception isn't?), but we actively discriminate between the ways or means to achieve it:

> A scheme of 'orientation in space' can be mediated relatively independently by visual, vestibular or proprioceptive channels.. . . . the subject can experience the co-existence of contradicting perceptions. When pushed to make a realistic appraisal of his orientation, the sensory channel(s) which, from experience, appear more veridical, are selected for the task (Bisdorff et al., 1996).

I wish the authors had used a different word than "veridical," which one can easily misread as "vertical." The point is clear nevertheless: we know "down" and "up" by visual cues, vestibular function, and by "haptic" sense or proprioception (Friedmann, 1970). If we require a realistic appraisal of the environment, we determine what seems true based on some kind of recalibration or "reweighting":

> . . . such re-weighting may be a requisite underlying compensation for the postural and perceptual effects of acute balance disorders . . ..

Sounds like a plan. But what about environmental tilts in which something's very obviously non-veridical in perception?

> This [re-weighting] scheme, however, may not apply to acute, focal brainstem lesions with marked lateropulsion, e.g. lateral medullary syndrome. In this case a tighter association between motor and perceptual aspects may exist, but only the SVV [subjective visual vertical], not the SPV [subjective postural vertical], has been measured in such patients. However . . . studies of the

visual vertical are not necessarily representative of other aspects of spatial orientation (Bisdorff et al., 1996).

I realize that I conflate thoughts about lateropulsion and sensations of environmental tilt. My rationale for doing so is to illuminate how awry the world can look in the context of lateral medullary disease. The lateral medulla, by the way, is where proprioceptive (lemniscal) and oculovestibular fibers are in intimate proximity. Consider the plain difficulty experienced by the one patient aware of his extreme lateropulsion–the one whose eyes "locked" to the right:

> The patient constantly preferred to keep his head turned to the left. In this way the eyes were kept in dextroversion when he looked at objects in front of him. He complained of a sensation of "locking the eyes" to the right, and attempted gaze to the left produced a definite feeling of discomfort which was difficult to verbalize distinctly. An increased sensation of instability of the visual field seemed to be a dominant feature (Hörnsten, 1974b).

Perhaps instability of the visual field reaches an apogee in cases of torsion of those fields.

*

If the subjective differs the from objective in any axis aside from vertical, a person wouldn't necessarily acknowledge any difference to herself, absent some frame of reference *like* the true gravitational vertical.

Hence the response "yup" to the woman whose eyes look subtly and conjugately askance from our examiner's vantage point?

The last sentence is meant to be a question, which you can cogitate at your leisure.

*

To come full circle, I recall that the answer book for the Residency In-Training Examination talked about how ocular lateropulsion in a lateral medullary syndrome is "likely due" to a lesion of olivocerebellar climbing fibers. I've since lost that book, which didn't reference the statement, if memory serves.

Maybe there are other answers aside from *a* lesion of olivocerebellar climbing fibers. What about a lesion of vestibular nuclei or of their many efferents in medulla or even in pons? Unless you're the patient herself, it's hard to be oblivious to ocular lateropulsion. The phenomenon begs questions about how we unconsciously represent the world relative to our own position and orientation in space.

14.

Canonical Medulla

By canonical, I mean an axial section of medulla in which we visualize all of the following together (in alphabetical order):

Ambiguus nucleus (related to CN IX and X),

Anterolateral fasciculus (a.k.a. spinothalamic tract),

Cochlear nuclei (CN VIII),

Descending tract and nucleus of CN V (a.k.a. spinal tract and nucleus of CN V),

Dorsal motor nucleus of Vagus (CN X),

Hypoglossal nucleus (CN XII),

Inferior cerebellar peduncle (a.k.a. restiform body– note that at our current level we visualize nothing of the brachium pontis or brachium conjunctivum; in other words, we are well caudal to the middle and superior cerebellar peduncles),

Inferior olive,

Medial lemniscus,

Medial longitudinal fasciculus,

Pyramid,

Solitary nucleus and tract (related to CN's VII, IX, and X),

Tectospinal tract, and

Vestibular nuclear column (CN VIII).

We've encountered the boldfaced items in past chapters. At the current level, it's relatively easy to organize the nuclei which we *haven't* yet visualized.

Applying a principle introduced in our chapter 4, we divide into alar/dorsal and basal/ventral based on sensory and motor nuclei, respectively. Where's the demarcation between alar/dorsal/sensory and basal/ventral/motor in medulla?

*

We require just two points to determine a line. I'll choose two that are noticeable: descending or spinal nucleus of CN V, which we've met in rostral cuts (see chapter 10), and solitary nucleus and tract (associated with CN's VII, IX, X), which is new to us. Solitary nucleus is hard to miss in atlases. Like the descending nucleus of CN V, solitary nucleus is located in the lateral medulla.

Draw a line along the under/ventral sides of spinal nucleus and of solitary nucleus. Extrapolate the line dorsally towards the floor of the fourth ventricle. The line points you directly at the **sulcus limitans** of Wilhelm His, Sr.

The sulcus limitans indents the fourth-ventricular floor just medial to the **vestibular triangle**. As we recall from chapter 10, the vestibular nuclei comprise a column that's present from medulla into pons, always lateral in its location in brainstem.

*

Nuclei derived from basal plate, **medial to the line**, including the **dorsal motor nucleus of Vagus** (CN X) and the **hypoglossal nucleus** (CN XII), are *motor*.

Nucleus ambiguus (related to CN IX and X) isn't easily seen in atlases, but its neurons are not ambiguously located. They're motor to soft palate, pharynx, and larynx. They're all medial to the line and dorsal to the principal nucleus of inferior olive.

If we move caudally towards the cervicomedullary junction, motor neurons contributing to the **spinal accessory nerve (CN XI)** are also medial to the line.

*

Nuclei derived from alar plate, **lateral to the line**, including the **solitary nucleus** and **sensory nucleus of CN V** themselves, the **vestibular nuclei** in the vestibular triangle, and **cochlear nuclei**, which drape themselves over the lateral aspect of the inferior cerebellar peduncles on either side, are *sensory*.

The solitary nucleus and tract receive fibers from CN's VII, IX, and X, related to taste (anterior 2/3 and posterior 1/3 of tongue) and visceral sensation from the heart, lungs, and gut.

Some facial sensory fibers (pinna and tragus of the ear) from CN VII and CN IX contribute to sensory nucleus and tract of CN V.

If we move caudally towards the cervicomedullary junction, sensory nuclei, such as the **gracile and cuneate nuclei**, are lateral to the line.

*

We're almost done, but strap in for the last mile or so of travel.

Teachers win points with students by way of their memory games. For the brainstem *as a whole*, for example (Gates, 2011), consider these four "rules," all conveniently related to the number 4:

> There are *four* structures in the midline starting with the letter M [Motor/corticospinal/pyramidal pathway, Medial lemnisci, Motor nuclei, Medial longitudinal fasciculus].
>
> There are *four* structures in the lateral brainstem starting with the letter S [Spinothalamic pathway, Sympathetic pathway, Sensory nucleus of the fifth cranial nerve, Spinocerebellar Tract].
>
> The lower *four* cranial nerves are in the medulla, the middle *four* are in the pons, and the first *four* cranial nerves are above the pons, with the third and fourth in the midbrain.
>
> The *four* motor cranial nerves that are in the midline are the four that divide evenly into 12 (except for 1 and 2)–that is, 3, 4, 6, and 12.

Two structures mentioned above have escaped discussion in this monograph: the Sympathetic pathway and Spinocerebellar tract. We won't ignore them, but we should acknowledge that they're tricky in anatomical terms. I've always enjoyed mnemonics of the sort just quoted, but my reason for liking them has changed over time. Today, for example, the riff on the number four makes me think harder about the actual anatomy.

There are two spinocerebellar tracts, first, a dorsal or posterior tract that feeds into inferior cerebellar peduncle without decussation across the midline. One doesn't see dorsal spinocerebellar tract above the medulla. Second, there's a ventral or anterior tract that can be found at all levels of lateral brainstem, but its route is roundabout. As with the dorsal tract, information transmitted has to do with unconscious proprioception (e.g., afferents from Golgi tendon organs in the limbs); decussation across the midline happens segmentally in spinal cord–for illustration, from right hemicord across to left–, then the tract ascends in the left lateral funiculus of cord, then lateral to (left) inferior olive in medulla, then lateral to the horizontally oriented (left) medial lemniscus in pons, then lateral to the (left) superior cerebellar peduncle at the pontomesencephalic border; fibers then cross the midline (they cross once again, now towards the right) in the decussation of the superior cerebellar peduncles en route to cerebellum. Is dorsal spinocerebellar tract lateral in medulla? Yes, only in medulla. Is ventral spinocerebellar tract lateral in medulla, pons, and midbrain? Nominally yes, but the second rule of 4 primarily addresses features of a lateral medullary syndrome.

In chapter 7, we mentioned but didn't fully discuss the sympathetic pathway within brainstem. I'll cut and paste to aid memory:

> . . . hypothalamic axons also descend in the **dorsal tegmental pathway**, although there's debate over whether, for example, projections from parvocelluluar paraventricular nucleus of hypothalamus connect monosynaptically with neurons in the spinal cord's intermediolateral grey column, from whence second-order arise in the sympathetic pupillodilatory pathway.

Dorsal tegmentum in low midbrain–tegmentum there is ventral to tectum, if you recall–refers us to the vicinity of CN IV (trochlear) nuclei, which stare at us a last time. First-order neurons in the sympathetic pathway aren't always lateral as they are in medulla. One way not to forget that anatomy is to think about a syndrome familiar to neuroophthalmologists: "The combination of an ipsilateral Horner syndrome (first-order) and contralateral superior oblique palsy (fourth nerve palsy) suggests a lesion of the trochlear nucleus or its fascicle in the brainstem" (Biousse and Newman, 2009). I trust that one understands why the palsy is contralateral to the lesion. One might also expect a head tilt towards the side of the superior oblique palsy, but the miosis/ptosis is on the same side as the low, paramedian mesencephalic lesion.

The first and second rules related to the number 4 address, for all intents and purposes, the demarcation between basal and alar plates best seen in the medulla. Those who teach about the sulcus limitans and the division of basal from alar, however, must confess what Nieuwenhuys himself called a limitation irrespective of the division's overall explanatory power. We need look no further than the inferior olive to be humbled.

The nucleus is of *alar plate origin*. So why is it medial to the line marked by our three landmarks (sulcus limitans at the floor of the fourth ventricle, the ventral side of solitary nucleus, the ventral side of spinal nucleus of CN V)?

Think even about the pons, where there is no inferior olive: pontine nuclei . . . are also of *alar plate origin* (Essick, 1912). So why are those alar entities, all those nuclei, so prominently located in the basis pontis?

The short answer is that the locations of inferior olive and pontine nuclei in adult human neuroanatomy are the consequence of lateral-to-medial tangential migrations during development.

Nieuwenhuys' work over many years, summarized in his 2011 paper, has informed this monograph from the start. As we end our tour, it seems there's new work to be done:

> . . . topological maps, derived from the brainstems of adult specimens, have certain important limitations, irrespective of their overall explanatory power. The exceptions discussed [e.g., inferior olive, pontine nuclei] make plain that the topological procedure does not project all cell masses back to their sites of origin and therewith to their primary topological positions. Conversely, it is now clear that the preparation of a *topological supermap*, showing the genuine primary positions of all constituent nuclei in the brainstem of a given species, would require

extensive neuroembryological studies, involving, *inter alia*, the expression patterns of numerous developmental regulatory genes and the tracing of all tangential migrations [author's emphasis].

A supermap? We'll stop quite shy of that.

15.

A Note on Brainstem Vasculature

From a 1961 paper, we read: "In a study of this type it is not sufficient merely to determine which of the large arteries is occluded–although previous authors have gone no further. A more exact delineation of the pattern of arterial distribution to the infarcted territory is necessary . . . " (Fisher et al., 1961). For 50 or so pages, he and his coauthors discuss vascular pathology affecting the lateral medulla. After a review of prior literature that starts the paper, they opine, "It would appear from this summary of the literature that the term 'posterior inferior cerebellar artery syndrome' was from the beginning a misnomer." Then the writing starts in earnest–a report of 16 cases of lateral medullary infarction, 14 of which had vascular occlusions, 12 of which had vertebral occlusions, and only 2 of which had occlusions of the posterior inferior cerebellar artery.

Many years ago, I had one encounter–my only contact, by phone–with the lead author. I had the sense that his was a medical intellect compared to which all others proved merely insufficient.

With his ghost in my head, what does one dare say about arteries to the entire brainstem? Like the approach throughout this monograph, I only offer aspects that have interested or helped me over time, all in the hope that the writing helps you, too.

As routine textbook chapters attest (Miyawaki, 2014), humans have the same larger arteries in the posterior circulation: vertebrals, basilar, superior cerebellar(s), and posterior cerebral(s). Vascular variability has to do with nuances regarding those large vessels as well as with the arteries of smaller caliber associated with them. For example, if the vertebrals aren't of the same caliber, then which is typically larger (the left one, perhaps)? If the left vertebral is larger, does the basilar tend to bend one way rather than the other (to the right, perhaps)? The anterior spinal artery is said to arise from both vertebrals, but where the two vertebrals fuse into the basilar is variable, so the level where the anterior spinal artery arises is also variable (Carpenter and Sutin, 1983). The origin the posterior inferior cerebellar artery is typically the vertebral, but proximal basilar is a variant; if the origin is the vertebral, sometimes the take-off of posterior inferior cerebellar artery is extradural, sometimes intradural. Not everyone has two anterior, inferior cerebellar arteries . . ..

Anatomical nuances are legion.

The reason why patterns of arterial distribution to an infarcted territory is important has to do with an inescapable fact that there's variation in the territories supplied by any given vessel, whether of larger or smaller caliber. And there's much overlap between arterial areas.

With the above in mind, and with preemptive apology to those of more encyclopedic bias, one can summarize the paramedian and circumferential supply of the brainstem at representative levels. The wedge-shaped approximate areas per axial level have indistinct or variable borders between them:

> In the hemi-medulla, from midline to lateral: territories of the **anterior spinal**, **vertebral**, and **posterior inferior cerebellar arteries**;

> In the mid-/hemi-pons, roughly at the level of the facial colliculi, from midline to lateral: territories of the **basilar** and **anterior inferior cerebellar arteries**;

In the upper hemi-pons, from midline to lateral: territories of the **basilar** and **superior cerebellar arteries**.

In the hemi-midbrain, from midline to lateral: territories of the **basilar** and **posterior cerebral arteries**.

Unilateral ischemic lesions abutting the midline seem reliably to obey it.

*

I'll conclude with case 5 from the 1961 series.

A 70 year-old woman had had problems with high blood pressure for three years prior to her presentation. Blood pressures ran roughly 190/100. Her only hypertensive symptom was occasional dizziness, about which we know little.

Six days prior to admission she experienced brief bouts of "weakness and dizziness."

Five days prior, she had a particularly severe attack in which she experienced a "spinning around" sensation. Her whole head hurt; she thought her left eye was out of focus.

Four days prior, she was "up and about," but still felt dizzy with a generalized headache. That afternoon, she found it difficult to swallow. She had double vision.

Three days prior, "intense numbness of the right face was added to the picture." One of her legs felt weak.

Two days prior, she occasionally saw objects "upside down." She continued to have problems swallowing. She felt restless.

By the time she presented to hospital, difficulty handling oral secretions had worsened; she often choked. Her speech was thick, with progression to speechlessness. She felt whole-body weakness.

On examination, she was febrile to 103° Fahrenheit and tachycardic (100 beats per minute). Blood pressure was 170/80 mmHg. Respirations were 15 per minute. She was cooperative, but unable to speak. Her pupils were small bilaterally, but both reacted to light and accommodation. There was nystagmus on upgaze, questionably so on lateral gaze. Sensation was diminished over the right face. Corneal reflexes were absent bilaterally. She had a left CN VI nerve palsy. She could not swallow. The tongue protruded weakly in the midline. She had a flaccid right hemiplegia. The left arm and leg moved slightly. Deep tendon reflexes were trace in the arms, save for a slightly greater right biceps reflex compared to the left. Knee and ankle jerks were absent. Both toes were extensor.

Her respirations slowed to five per minute. Stupor followed. She died on the second house day (Fisher et al., 1961).

*

The pace of the story, never mind the ending, disturbs.

Since we know that all 16 cases of the series involved infarction of the lateral medulla, questions arise.

1. When did hers occur?
2. On day 5 prior to admission, what's to be made of her left eye being out of focus? Do we discard the information, because it's monocular? Answer: we could, but the series referenced in chapter 13 (Hörnsten, 1974) describes such monocular symptoms. Why, then, the left eye?
3. Did hers occur when the swallowing difficulty commenced (4 days prior to admission)?
4. On day 3 prior to admission, does the addition of the right face numbness cinch a medullary localization? If so, what's to be made of the weakness in one of her legs?
5. If you discount the weakness on day 3, then what's to be made of the flaccid right hemiplegia in her examination on the day of admission?
6. Two days prior, when she occasionally saw the world upside down, was that when her stroke happened or were the sensations of environmental tilt epiphenomena?

7. In the reported examination, why were both pupils small and why were corneal reflexes absent *bilaterally*?
8. Regarding the left CN VI palsy, we recall from chapter 10 that if the lesion were nuclear, we'd rather expect a left facial palsy and an associate conjugate gaze palsy (to the left), but we see neither.
9. If you invoke a lesion of left paramedian pontine reticular formation, how does the exam not corroborate your thought? Answer: if paramedian pontine reticular formation, wouldn't you expect a conjugate gaze palsy to the left (*both* eyes unable to look leftward)?
10. Why were both toes extensor?
11. Why the stupor?

You're eager for answers. I understand.

Recall, though, that the motivation for *Learning the Brainstem* was to get you to think like a local for yourself. The authors themselves don't rush in with answers to the 11 or many more questions that you could ask about the 70 year-old woman:

> This case is an example of the lateral medullary syndrome associated with thrombosis of the right VA [vertebral artery], and accompanied by a separate pontine infarct. [On review of the pathology,] the lateral medullary infarct at the mid-olivary level accounted for most of the patient's prodromal and early manifestations. The vessel of supply to the region of the medullary infarct was identified as a branch of the VA [vertebral artery]. This case illustrates that the [lateral medullary] syndrome is not always benign, but can presage a basilar artery thrombosis if the involved VA [vertebral artery] is the only adequate source of supply to the basilar territory. Damage to the brainstem was likely more extensive than portrayed in the stained

[pathological] section since the pontine lesion could not have accounted for the stupor or the 6th nerve palsy (Fisher et al., 1961).

Welcome to an honest case in which you have to think *through* your fundamental three choices. The brainstem, healthy or not, will be found in your clinical examination.

References

Books and monographs

Biousse, Valérie and Newman, Nancy J. *Neuro-ophthalmology Illustrated.* New York and Stuttgart: Thieme, 2009.

Brazis, Paul W., Masdeu, Joseph C., and Biller, José. *Localization in Clinical Neurology.* Boston and Toronto: Little, Brown, 1985.

Brodal, A. *Neurological Anatomy In Relation to Clinical Medicine.* [3rd ed.] New York and Oxford: Oxford University Press, 1981.

Carpenter, Malcolm B. and Sutin, Jerome. *Human Neuroanatomy.* [8th ed.] Baltimore and London: Williams and Wilkins, 1983.

Cordo, Paul and Harnad, Stevan, eds. *Movement Control.* New York: Cambridge University Press, 1994.

DeArmond, Stephen J., Fusco, Madeline M., and Dewey, Maynard M. *Structure of the Human Brain. A Photographic Atlas.* [3rd ed.] New York, Oxford: Oxford University Press, 1989.

Glaser, Joel S., ed. *Neuro-ophthalmology.* [2nd ed.] Philadelphia: J.B. Lippincott, 1990.

Kahle, Werner. *Nervous system and Sensory Organs.* [3rd revised ed., trans. H.L. and A.D. Dayan, Volume 3 of Kahle W., Leonhardt H, Platzer W. *Color Atlas and Textbook of Human Anatomy*] Stuttgart and New York: Georg Thieme, 1986.

Llinás, Rodolfo R. *I of the Vortex. From Neurons to Self.* Cambridge and London: MIT Press, 2001.

Miyawaki, Edison K. *The Crossed Organization of Brains*. Bloomington: Xlibris, 2018a.

Miyawaki, Edison K. *The Frontal Brain and Language*. Bloomington: Xlibris, 2018b.

Nauta, Walle J.H. and Feirtag, Michael. *Fundamental Neuroanatomy*. New York: W.H. Freeman, 1986.

Nieuwenhuys, Rudolf. *Chemoarchitecture of the Brain*. Berlin/Heidelberg/New York/Tokyo: Springer Verlag, 1985.

Nieuwenhuys, Rudolf, Voogd, Jan, and van Huijzen, Christiaan. *The Human Central Nervous System*. Fourth ed. Berlin/Heidelberg/New York: Springer Verlag, 2008.

Nolte, John. *The Human Brain. An Introduction to Its Functional Anatomy*. [4th ed.] St. Louis: Mosby, 1999.

Shepherd, Gordon M., ed. *The Synaptic Organization of the Brain* [4th ed]. New York and Oxford: Oxford University Press, 1998.

Swanson, Larry W. *Neuroanatomical Terminology. A Lexicon of Classical Origins and Historical Foundations*. Oxford and New York: Oxford University Press, 2015.

*

Articles, Specific Chapters in Books

Alexander GE, DeLong MR, Crutcher MD. Naturalizing motor control theory: isn't it time for a new paradigm? In: *Movement Control*. Eds. Cordo, P and Harnard, S. Cambridge: Cambridge University Press, 1994, pp. 226-231.

Aravamuthan BR, Muthusamy KA, Stein JF, Aziz TZ, Johansen-Berg H. Topography of cortical and subcortical connections of the human pedunculopontine and subthalamic nuclei. *NeuroImage* 2007;37:694-705.

Bahsi I, Orhan M, Kervancioglu P, Bahsi A. Constanzo Varolio (1543-1575), who named the "pons." *Child's Nervous System* 2018;34:585-588.

Baizer JS, Sherwood CC, Hof PR, Witelson SF, Sultan F. Neurochemical and structural organization of the principal nucleus of the inferior olive in the human. *The Anatomical Record* 2011;294:1198-1216.

Bisdorff AR, Wolsley CJ, Anastasopoulos D, Bronstein AM, Gresty MA. The perception of body verticality (subjective postural vertical) in peripheral and central vestibular disorders. *Brain* 1996;119:1523-1534.

Blomfield S and Marr D. How the cerebellum may be used. *Nature* 1970;227:1224-1228.

Brazis PW. The localization of lesions affecting the brainstem. In: *Localization in Clinical Neurology*. Eds. Brazis PW, Masdeu JC, Biller J. Boston and Toronto: Little, Brown, 1985, pp. 225-238.

Broga C, Fiengo L, Türe U. Achille Louis Foville's atlas of brain anatomy and Defoville syndrome. *Neurosurgery* 2012;70:1265-1273.

Bronstein AM, Pérennou DA, Guerraz M, Playford D, Rudge P. Dissociation of visual and haptic vertical in two patients with vestibular nuclear lesions. *Neurology* 2003;61:1260-1262.

Burnstock G. Autonomic neurotransmission: 60 years since Sir Henry Dale. *Annual Review of Pharmacology and Toxicology* 2009;49:1-30.

Büttner-Ennever JA. The extraocular motor nuclei: organization and functional neuroanatomy. *Progress in Brain Research* 2006;151:95-125.

Carpenter MB and Pierson RJ. Pretectal region and the pupillary light reflex. An anatomical analysis in the monkey. *Journal of Comparative Neurology* 1973;149:271-300.

Chandrasekhar A. Turning heads: development of vertebrate branchiomotor neurons. *Developmental Dynamics* 2004;229:143-161.

Chandraskehar A, Moens CB, Warren JT, Kimmel CB, Kuwada JY. Development of branchiomotor neurons in zebrafish. *Development* 1997;124:2633-2644.

Coenen VA, Schumacher LV, Kaller C, Schlaepfer TE, Reinacher PC, Egger K, Urbach H, Reisert M. The anatomy of the human medial forebrain bundle: ventral tegmental area connections to reward-associated subcortical and frontal lobe regions. *NeuroImage: Clinical* 2018;18:770-783.

Cohen B, Komatsuzaki A, Bender MB. Electrooculographic syndrome in monkeys after pontine reticular formation lesions. *Archives of Neurology* 1968;18:78-92.

Cooper ERA. The trochlear nerve in the human embryo and foetus. *British Journal of Ophthalmology* 1947;31:257-75.

Daroff RB, Troost BT, Leigh RJ. Supranuclear disorders of eye movements. In: *Neuro-ophthalmology* [2nd ed.]. Ed. Glaser JS. Philadelphia: J.B. Lippincott, 1990, pp. 299-323.

Davidoff RA, Atkin A, Anderson PJ, Bender MB. Optokinetic nystagmus and cerebral disease. Clinical and pathological study. *Archives of Neurology* 1966;14:73-81.

Dieterich M and Brandt T. Ocular torsion and tilt of subjective vertical are sensitive brainstem signs. *Annals of Neurology* 1993;33:292-299.

Essick CR. The development of the nuclei pontis and the nucleus arcuatus in man. *American Journal of Anatomy* 1912;13:25-54.

Fisher CM. Ataxic hemiparesis. A pathologic study. *Archives of Neurology* 1978;35:126-128.

Fisher CM and Cole M. Homolateral ataxia and crural paresis: a vascular syndrome. *Journal of Neurology, Neurosurgery, and Psychiatry* 1965;28:48-55.

Fisher CM, Karnes WE, Kubik CS. Lateral medullary infarction– the pattern of vascular occlusion. *Journal of Neuropathology and Experimental Neurology* 1961;20:323-379.

Foville A. Note sur une paralysie peu connue de certains muscles de l'œil, et sa liaison avec quelques points de l'anatomie et la physiologie de la protubérance annulaire. *Bulletins de la Société Anatomique de Paris* 1858;33:393-414.

Friedmann G. The judgement of the visual vertical and horizontal with peripheral and central vestibular lesions. *Brain* 1970;93:313-328.

Fritzsch B. Of mice and genes: evolution of vertebrate brain development. *Brain, Behavior and Evolution* 1998;52:207-217.

Frohman TC, Galetta S, Fox R, Solomon D, Straumann D, Filippi M, Zee D, Frohman EM. Pearls and Oy-sters: the medial longitudinal fasciculus in ocular motor physiology. *Neurology* 2008;70:e57-e67.

Fukushima K. The interstitial nucleus of Cajal and its role in the control of movements of head and eyes. *Progress in Neurobiology* 1987;29:107-192.

Gates P. Work out where the problem is in the brainstem using 'the rule of 4.' *Practical Neurology* 2011;11:167-172.

Gautier JC and Blackwood W. Enlargement of the inferior olivary nucleus in association with lesions of the central tegmental tract or dentate nucleus. *Brain* 1961;84:341-361.

Goldman-Rakic PS. The "psychic" neuron of the cerebral cortex. *Annals of the New York Academy of Sciences* 1999;868:13-26.

Hartline PH. Physiological basis for detection of sound and vibration in snakes. *Journal of Experimental Biology* 1971;54:349-371.

Haubenberger D and Hallett M. Essential tremor. *New England Journal of Medicine* 2018;378:1802-1809.

Hikosaka O. The habenula: from stress evasion to value-based decision-making. *Nature Reviews Neuroscience* 2010;11:503-513.

Hikosaka O, Takikawa Y, Kawagoe R. Role of the basal ganglia in the control of purposive saccadic eye movements. *Physiological Reviews* 2000;80:953-978.

Hörnsten G. Wallenberg's syndrome. Part I. General symptomatology, with special reference to visual disturbances and imbalance. *Acta Neurologica Scandinavica* 1974(a);50:434-446.

Hörnsten G. Wallenberg's syndrome. Part II. Oculomotor and oculostatic disturbances. *Acta Neurologica Scandinavica* 1974(b);50:447-468.

Irving R and Harrison JM. The superior olivary complex and audition: a comparative study. *Journal of Comparative Neurology* 1967;130:77-86.

Jones EG. Golgi, Cajal and the neuron doctrine. *Journal of the History of the Neurosciences* 1999;8:170-178.

Kinney HC, Broadbelt KG, Haynes RL, Rognum IJ, Paterson DS. The serotonergic anatomy of the developing human medulla oblongata: implications for pediatric disorders of homeostasis. *Journal of Chemical Neuroanatomy* 2011;41:182-199.

Kinney HC and Samuels MA. Neuropathology of the persistent vegetative state. A review. *Journal of Neuropathology and Experimental Neurology* 1994;53:548-558.

Lapresle J and Hamida MB. The dentato-olivary pathway. Somatotopic relationship between the dental nucleus and the contralateral inferior olive. *Archives of Neurology* 1970;22:135-143.

Longetti P, Fiorindi A, Feletti A, D'Avella D, Martinuzzi A. Endoscopic anatomy of the fourth ventricle. Laboratory investigation. *Journal of Neurosurgery* 2008;109:530-555.

Marx JJ, Iannetti GD, Thömke F, Fitzek S, Urban PP, Stoeter P, Cruccu G, Dieterich M, Hopf HC. Somatotopic organization of the corticospinal tract in the human brainstem: a MRI-based mapping analysis. *Annals of Neurology* 2005;57:824-831.

Mastick GS and Easter SS. Initial organization of neurons and tracts in the embryonic mouse fore- and midbrain. *Developmental Biology* 1996;173:79-94.

May PJ, Reiner AJ, Ryabinin AE. Comparison of the distributions of urocortin-containing and cholinergic neurons in the perioculomotor midbrain of the cat and macaque. *Journal of Comparative Neurology* 2008;507:1300-1316.

McCrea RA and Baker R. Anatomical connections of the nucleus prepositus of the cat. *Journal of Comparative Neurology* 1985;237:377-407.

McCrea RA and Horn AKE. Nucleus prepositus. *Progress in Brain Research* 2006;151:205-230.

McKay IJ, Lewis J, Lumsden A. Organization and development of facial motor neurons in the *Kreisler* mutant mouse. *European Journal of Neuroscience* 1997;9:1499-1506.

Miyawaki EK. Cerebral Arteries. In: Aminoff MJ and Daroff RB, eds. *Encyclopedia of the Neurological Sciences* [2nd ed.]. Oxford: Academic Press, 2014, pp. 651-657.

Moore JK. The human auditory brain stem: a comparative view. *Hearing Research* 1987;29:1-32.

Moore RY and Bloom FE. Central catecholamine neuron systems: anatomy and physiology of the dopamine systems. *Annual Review of Neuroscience* 1978;1:129-169.

Moreno-Bravo JA, Martinez-Lopez JE, Puelles E. Review. Mesencephalic neuronal populations. New insights on the ventral differentiation programs. *Histology and Histopathology* 2012;27:1529-1538.

Müller F, O'Rahilly R. The development of the human brain, including the longitudinal zoning in the diencephalon at stage 15. *Anatomy and Embryology* 1988;179:55-71.

Müller F, O'Rahilly R. The initial appearance of the cranial nerves and related neuronal migration in staged human embryos. *Cells Tissues Organs* 2011;193:215-238.

Nakamura H. Regionalization of the optic tectum: combinations of gene expression that define the tectum. *Trends in Neurosciences* 2001;24:32-39.

Nathan PW and Smith MC. The rubrospinal and central tegmental tracts in man. *Brain* 1982;105:223-269.

Ngwa EC, Zeeh C, Messoudi A, Büttner-Ennever JA, Horn AKE. Delineation of motoneuron subgroups supplying individual eye muscles in the human oculomotor nucleus. *Frontiers in Neuroanatomy* 2014;8:article 2, doi: 10.3389/fnana.2014.00002.

Nieuwenhuys R. The structural, functional, and molecular organization of the brainstem. *Frontiers in Neuroanatomy* 2011;5:article 33, doi: 10.3389/fnana.2011.00033.

Ohtsuka K and Nagasaka Y. Divergent axon collaterals from the rostral superior colliculus to the pretectal accommodation-related areas and the omnipause neuron area in the cat. *Journal of Comparative Neurology* 1999;413:68-76.

Pombal MA, Megías M. Development and functional organization of the cranial nerves in lampreys. *The Anatomical Record* 2018; doi: 10.1002/ar.23821.

Puelles K, Tvrdik P, Martínez-De-La-Torre M. The postmigratory alar topography of visceral cranial nerve efferents challenges the classical model of hindbrain columns. *The Anatomical Record* 2018 Apr 16, doi: 10.1002/ar.23830.

Rakic P. A small step for the cell, a giant leap for mankind: a hypothesis of neocortical expansion during evolution. *Trends in Neurosciences* 1995;18:383-388.

Rasmussen AT and Peyton WT. Origin of the ventral external arcuate fibers and their continuity with the striae medullares of the fourth ventricle of man. *The Anatomical Record* 1946;84:325-337.

Ruigrok TJH and Voogd J. Organization of projections from the inferior olive to the cerebellar nuclei in the rat. *Journal of Comparative Neurology* 2000;426:209-228.

Salma A, Yeremeyeva E, Baidya NB, Sayers MP, Ammirati M. Neuroanatomical study. An endoscopic, cadaveric analysis of the roof of the fourth ventricle. *Journal of Clinical Neuroscience* 2013;20:710-714.

Sato T, Joyner AL, Nakamura H. Review. How does FgF signaling from the isthmic organizer induce midbrain and cerebellar development? *Development, Growth, and Differentiation* 2004;46:487-494.

Schmahmann JD, Ko R, MacMore J. The human basis pontis: motor syndromes and topographic organization. *Brain* 2004;127:1269-1291.

Selvadurai C, Rondeau MW, Colorado RA, Feske SK, Prasad S. Teaching video Neuro*Images*: Foville syndrome. *Neurology* 2016;86:e203.

Sharpe JA. What's up, doc? Altered perception of the haptic, postural, and visual vertical. *Neurology* 2003;61:1172-1173.

Shute CCD and Lewis PR. The ascending cholinergic reticular system: neocortical, olfactory and subcortical projections. *Brain* 1967;90:497-520.

Sierra-Hidalgo F, de Pablo-Fernández E, Herrero-San Martin A, Correas-Callero E, Herreros-Rodríguez J, Romero-Muñoz JP, Martín-Gil L. Clinical and imaging features of the room tilt illusion. *Journal of Neurology* 2012;259:2555-2564.

Silverman IE, Liu GT, Volpe NJ, Galetta SL. The crossed paralyses. The original brain-stem syndromes of Millard-Gubler, Foville, Weber, and Raymond-Cestan. *Archives of Neurology* 1995;52:635-638.

Sterling P. Retina. In: *The Synaptic Organization of the Brain*. Ed. Shepherd GM. New York: Oxford, 1998, see especially p. 225.

Voogd J, van Baarsen K. The horseshoe-shaped commissure of Wernekinck or the decussation of the brachium conjunctivum. Methodological changes in the 1840's. *Cerebellum* 2014;13:113-120.

Zec N, Filiano JJ, Kinney HC. Anatomic relationships of the human arcuate nucleus of the medulla; a DiI-labeling study. *Journal of Neuropathology and Experimental Neurology* 1997;56:509-522.

www.ingramcontent.com/pod-product-compliance
Lightning Source LLC
Chambersburg PA
CBHW021442210526
45463CB00002B/616